The Homeopathic Treatment of
Depression, Anxiety, Bipolar Disorder
and other
Mental and Emotional Problems

To our patients, who have placed their trust in us and have taught us so much about the human psyche and spirit. We wish for them, and for all other beings, happiness and peace.

The Homeopathic Treatment of Depression, Anxiety, Bipolar Disorder and other Mental and Emotional Problems

Homeopathic Alternatives to Conventional Drug Therapies

Judyth Reichenberg-Ullman, N.D., M.S.W.
Robert Ullman, N.D.

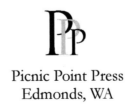

Picnic Point Press
Edmonds, WA

This book is intended for education purposes only. It is not intended to diagnose, treat, or give medical advice for aspecific condition, or to in any way replace the services of a qualified medical practitioner.

The cases in this book are true stories from the authors' clinical practice. The names of the patents have been changed to protect confidentiality. Any names matching or resembling those of real people are coincidental and unintentional.

Previously Published as Prozac-Free
by Crown Publishing Group 1999,
and North Atlantic Books, 2002
First Revised English Edition 2012
© Judyth Reichenberg-Ullman, N.D., M.S.W. and Robert Ullman, N.D.
Picnic Point Press, 2012

Printed in the United States of America

Library of Congress Cataloging-in-Publication Data

Reichenberg-Ullman, Judyth.
      The homeopathic treatment of depression, anxiety, bipolar disorder and other mental and emotional problems : homeopathic alternatives to conventional drug therapies / Judyth Reichenberg-Ullman, Robert Ullman. -- 1st Rev. English ed.
          p. cm.
      Previously published: Prozac-free/Judyth Reichenberg-Ullman, Robert Ullman. c2002.
      Includes bibliographical references and index.
      ISBN 978-0-9640654-0-6 (trade pbk.)
      1. Depression, Mental--Homeopathic treatment. 2. Mental illness--Homeopathic treatment. 3. Mental illness--Alternative treatment. I. Ullman, Robert. II. Reichenberg-Ullman, Judyth. Prozac-free. III. Title.

RX301.M45.R447 2012
615.5'32--dc23

2012003737

Contents

Foreword

This revised edition of *Prozac Free* is indeed a most welcome and needed addition to the growing number of homeopathic books published in recent years. *Prozac Free* and *Ritalin-Free Kids*, the Ullmans' previous bestseller, are among the best books that focus exclusively on the psychiatric applications of homeopathy.

Judyth Reichenberg-Ullman and Robert Ullman are the perfect people to write this book. Licensed naturopathic physicians board-certified in homeopathic medicine, they bring to their readers over thirty years of experience as homeopaths, as well as over thirty-five years as mental health professionals. I met Judyth and Robert at the beginning of their careers in homeopathy and at the same time that they met each other. Since then they have become among the best known and respected authors and teachers in the North American homeopathic community. They have a special talent for sharing their knowledge and love of homeopathy in a down-to-earth, easy-to-understand style. The Ullmans' mission is to make homeopathy accessible, comprehensible and available to the general public and the professional community as well as to raise the standards of homeopathic education and practice.

I am a psychiatrist and homeopath. I am called often by those wishing to know if this or that mental or emotional problem — their own or that of a family member or friend — can be helped by homeopathy. Is there a recommended book that can be read prior to making an appointment? Unfortunately, until now, I have had to recommend books that are not quite suitable. Finally a book has been written to which I can refer those seeking alternatives to psychiatric pharmaceutical drugs, and I have been given the honor of writing its foreword.

The case histories which comprise the largest portion of this book are wonderful examples of how homeopathy has helped people with mental, emotional, behavioral, and personality disorders. To the reader with no prior experience with homeopathy, the cases presented may seem implausibly miraculous. Results like these with harmless, highly dilute medicines? Yes. If we could ask other well-trained, experienced homeopaths if they also see these kinds of results, every one of them would say, "Yes, this is what happens when you give the correct homeopathic medicine." In my thirty years as a psychiatrist I have found over and over again that nothing can match homeopathy in efficacy for treating mental and emotional illness when the provider of homeopathic treatment is a well-trained and competent classical homeopath.

Why has it taken so long for homeopathy to break out of the fringes of medicine into the mainstream in the United States when it is already an acknowledged medical art in Europe, Latin America and India? The reasons are undoubtedly complex. One might say that no movement can enter the cultural mainstream which is itself not compatible with the spirit of the times, the Zeitgeist. An excessively strong materialistic bias in American science and medicine has been a big factor. The weakening of the death-grip which mechanistic materialism has had on the scientific and intellectual community coupled with the growing popularity of vitalistic ideas has allowed homeopathy to come out of isolation. And, incredibly, at the same time homeopathy has been blessed by the world-wide emergence of brilliant teachers. This has allowed many contemporary classical homeopaths to broaden and deepen their knowledge at an astonishingly rapid pace and to aspire to (and obtain) excellent results like those described by the Ullmans in their books. This book draws wonderfully on the "new homeo-pathy", if I may coin a phrase to distinguish it from nineteenth century theory and practice, in its deep and penetrating insight into patients and in discerning the appropriate medicines for them.

The new homeopathy probes with great depth and accuracy into the nitty gritty of the patient's difficulties. The reader may note that there is no psychiatric or psychological jargon in the homeopathic analysis. The patient is described and understood in his or her own terms. One must understand the patient correctly and in-depth based on what one hears and sees. The patient's suffering must be translated into the language of homeopathy in order to find a correct medicine. The homeopath must honor the patient's unique expression of self. Doing otherwise is to flirt with failure.

Although homeopathy can produce dramatic results with many psychiatric patients, let's not toss out the baby with the bath water. As a medical doctor, psychiatrist and homeopath, I haven't thrown away my prescription pad. Psychopharmaceutical drugs remain indispensable in many situations. Though my preference is to use homeopathy for every patient, the concurrent, continued use of prescription medications may be necessary, at least temporarily and sometimes permanently. Even in those cases where we cannot take the patient off psychiatric drugs, we usually can reduce the dosage and thereby decrease uncomfortable side effects, while at the same time producing real improvements in functioning.

Homeopathic treatment of mental and emotional disorders characteristically results in an increase in vitality, self-perception, self-knowledge and feelings of well-being. Homeopathy, if practised on a wide scale, has great promise as a social psychiatry. If practised in the prison system, recidivism could be greatly decreased. Perpetrators and victims of domestic violence respond well to homeopathic treatment. The antisocial behaviors of those adolescents and children who disrupt the classroom could be eliminated if homeopathy were as easily available as Ritalin. One needs merely to extrapolate from the remarkable case histories presented in this book to imagine the possibilities for social transformation with the widespread application of homeopathy to the mental, emotional and personality disorders that are the direct and indirect causes of most of the unhappiness on our planet.

This book is far more than an introduction to psychiatric homeopathy. Professional homeopaths will find it immensely useful and stimulating; the authors have presented many unusual medicines which are straight from the cutting edge of the theory and practice of the new homeopathy. Psychiatrists, psychologists, social workers and other psychotherapists may discover an alternative to conventional drugs for those of their clientele who need medication. Homeopathic treatment does not replace psychotherapy. Psychotherapists who refer to homeopaths will not only be astonished by the relief of distress afforded by homeopathic treatment but pleased by the enhancement of therapy. Homeopathy results in increased self-perception and deeper insight which enables therapy to progress far more rapidly and effectively. These remarkable medicines seem to break the "resistance" to therapy. Homeopathic treatment removes depression, anxiety, delusions, dissociation and other symptoms so that therapy can do what it really does best: promote growth and development through self knowledge.

Homeopathy is a gift for those who wish to understand themselves more deeply, remove negativity, and live more expansively in love and creativity. Homeopathy, exquisitely gentle yet incredibly powerful, is for those who understand that the golden hammer opens the iron door.

Michael K. Glass, M.D.

Ithaca, New York

Acknowledgments

We thank our teachers, particularly Dr. Rajan Sankaran, who has informed, inspired, and revitalized our homeopathic practice since we began studying with him in 1993. It is thanks to his brilliant guidance that we have been able to prescribe medicines we had never considered, or even known of, with such dramatic results.

Introduction

A Better Answer for a Happier World

We do not live in a happy society. An astounding number of individuals rely on prescription medication, as you will see as you read further in our book, to keep their thoughts positive and their moods stable. Contemporary, highly technological life is complex, fast-moving, quickly changing and highly unpredictable. The common wisdom is that it is necessary, simply a matter of course, to take pharmaceutical uppers, downers, or whatever is needed to remain on an even keel. What if we told you that there is another type of medicine, one that is safe, long-lasting, deep-acting, highly affective, and has the potential to alleviate your physical problems as well as your depression? A medicine that is inexpensive, individualized to your unique symptoms, and one which you need to take only infrequently. One that produces significant positive changes with more frequency than Prozac or other conventional medications. And what if we shared with you the true experiences of others who were depressed but who now feel very well thanks to this medicine? Would you consider a different alternative? We hope so! This is our reason for writing this book and has been the career to which we have dedicated ourselves over the past thirty years.

Who are we to dare to suggest a natural alternative to antidepressants, especially at a time when many think that serotonin-regulating drugs are the panacea for mood disorders? We are licensed naturopathic physicians board-certified in homeopathic medicine. From 1976 to 1978 Judyth was a psychiatric social worker assigned to the locked psychiatric ward of a major teaching hospital, in halfway houses, outpatient clinics and private homes. Robert has worked extensively with hospitalized psychiatric patients and developmentally-disabled children and adults. Disillusioned by the side effects and partial and temporary improvement resulting from major tranquilizers and other psychiatric medications compounded with numerous, often serious, side effects, we became convinced that there must be a gentler and more effective solution to mental illness. Each of us came to this realization a decade before we ever met each other.

As you can see from the many patients we have treated successfully whose cases we recount in our book, we believe we have found an answer that can transform the lives of many people. We present these real, but anonymous, cases from our practice and ask you to draw your own conclusions about the effectiveness of homeopathy.

Val's Success with Homeopathic Treatment for Depression

Let us share with you the story of Val, one of thousands of patients with mental and emotional problems that we have treated over the past fifteen years. A computer programmer from Eastern Washington, Val was 38 years old when she first came to our clinic nine years ago. Discouraged and disappointed, after having put on thirty extra pounds, Val simply wanted to feel better. A starvation diet through a weight loss clinic and four mile a day walks five days a week had not been enough to shed the excess weight.

Val suffered great annoyance from her environmental and food allergies, which caused a myriad of symptoms including dizziness, a seriously stuffy nose, irritability, bloating, migraines and 4 A.M. panic attacks. Annoyance crossed over the line to misery during the spring and fall hay fever seasons when her headaches, sneezing and dizziness were constant. At the age of two, Val, never having been breast-fed, was covered with eczema from head to toe due to her sensitivity to cow's milk. Dry, chapped, bleeding, cracked skin still bothered her with some frequency. She also complained of ringing in her ears, athlete's foot, heartburn, premenstrual headaches, constipation and offensive body odor. You can easily understand why Val wanted to find a way to feel better.

"I've been depressed as long as I can remember," she shared with us. "I've had suicidal feelings about twice a month for years. I guess I take after my mother who was on antidepressants for thirty years." Val had not realized her dream of writing children's books. She had contemplated relocating to a different city, a career change, moving to a different apartment.

Nothing she tried, including years of psychotherapy focusing on her dysfunctional family, had really made a difference. Val described her father as responsible but absent and her mother as a tyrant. A quiet child, she coped by becoming "lost in a dream world with a cast of thousands". A sensitive peacemaker, Val proved herself by achieving straight A's, being the class valedictorian, and by completing two graduate degrees. As a "loner egghead", friendships did not come easily. Nor did intimate relationships except when she fantasized about movie stars and guitar heroes. Despite her quick wit, vivid imagination, and pleasant personality, Val was unable to make deep connections with others.

Val had a nervous streak, even as an adolescent. In college her worries escalated into full-blown anxiety attacks. Uncomfortable in tight places, she preferred to wait for an empty elevator.

Val benefitted considerably from *Aurum sulphuricum* (gold sulfide). Her moods, allergies, heartburn, headaches, abdominal distress, dizziness, athlete's foot, explosive diarrhea, eczema, sinusitis and body odor all improved significantly. Others told her that she looked better. Her anxiety was much reduced and she felt more stable emotionally. We prescribed a dose of the medicine on an average of once every four to six months.

As we came to know and understand her better, Val confided that her biggest issues were despair about feeling she had failed in her career, doubt of her ability to survive, and a disconnectedness from others. After four years of periodic visits, Val described herself as "happier than I've been in years. I'm back to writing and researching. I have no suicidal thoughts. I get up in the morning and I'm happy to be alive. I'm amazed. I'm feeling so much better emotionally. I'm sleeping well and I'm having no anxiety attacks."

As homeopaths do, we continually tried to delve more deeply into Val's state. "Part of my problem in defining myself", she shared, "is that I don't know what I feel. In childhood I learned not even to think. I didn't really develop an identity until I was in college." She also mentioned her terrible constipation as a child. This led to finely tune the medicine even further to *Aluminum sulphuricum* (aluminum sulfate), which has been repeated four times over the past 14 months. An excellent medicine for people who lack a clear sense of self and self-control, often as a result of being raised by a dominant parent who suppressed the child's will and individuality, this medicine also matched Val's physical symptoms very well.

Val has continued to feel progressively better. She now owns a home, which allows her to feel comfortable and secure, and is more satisfied with her work. Generally even-tempered and on an even keel, she continues to feel quite well rather than "lost in the trough" as she did prior to homeopathic treatment. She is spending more creative time on her writing and still hopes to publish her work. Val continues to work on herself and, although her life is not perfect, it is dramatically improved from when we started working together and she has not needed to resort to antidepressants. Yes, there *is* happiness and well-being without drugs. You will read many stories in our book about people who, like Val, have experienced wonderful changes in their lives from homeopathy.

What Makes YOU Tick?

Despite all the scientific research regarding serotonin and other neurotransmitters, we, as homeopaths, do not believe that the human mind or body can be wrapped up into a neat little package. Given so many different manifestations and variations on unhappiness, it does not make sense to us that they can all be attributed to one cause.

Conventional wisdom in mainstream medicine is habituated to finding a finite number of categorical boxes into which you can potentially be placed. If you can be pigeonholed into a diagnostic box, then your doctor can find the medicine or medicines that correspond.

The problem, to our way of thinking and our clinical experience, is that this approach misses entirely the inherent uniqueness and individuality of each human being. By trying to find commonalities in people and symptoms, you might be able to narrow them down to half a dozen or fewer possible medications. The problem is that the more specialized conventional medicine has become, the more you are likely to be evaluated in pieces rather than as a whole, integrated human being.

A homeopathic practitioner, to the contrary, tries to discover just what makes you tick and why you became depressed in the first place. We do not try to fit people into a narrow range of diagnostic categories in order to prescribe one of a handful of medicines. We listen to your story, understanding that, in its own way, it is unlike any story we have every heard before, then we prescribe for you as an individual, one of nearly two thousand safe and natural homeopathic medicines.

Some of you may be perfectly satisfied taking antidepressants but we know that many of you chose to read this book because you are seeking a safe and effective alternative. We hope that it will inspire you to open your mind to another alternative, one that might bring you and others you know and love more far-reaching and lasting healing than antidepressants. Homeopathy is fascinating and complex. To prescribe effectively for depression and other serious mental and emotional problems requires years of training and experience. Homeopathy, like any type of medicine, cannot help everyone, but we estimate that a well-trained and experienced homeopathic physician or practitioner can help up to 70% of those who are committed to continuing treatment for at least one year. You are likely to begin to feel better within four to six weeks of beginning treatment, sometimes sooner.

If you choose to pursue homeopathy for yourself or your loved ones, do not even consider prescribing for yourself. Find a practitioner who is well-trained, highly-qualified and experienced as a homeopath, as well as seasoned in treating patients with mental and emotional issues, to help you. Then, you will be more likely to experience the positive results that we discuss in our book. Regardless of which path you choose, we wish you the very best with healing and hope that you find happiness and peace.

However, homeopathy is not a quick fix, but rather a deep healing process that unfolds over time. Although you will be aware of some physical, mental, and emotional shifts within a matter of weeks or months, it is important to continue homeopathic care. Over one to five years, not only will symptoms be alleviated, but the fundamental underlying state will change as well. This is often a state that was acquired, as a result of trauma, illness, life experience or events, and was frozen into a persistent condition . Although it does not serve the individual, and, in fact, contributes to the imbalance, disease, and unhappiness, it persists, often lifelong. Homeopathic treatment can, with great benefit, produce such a profound shift that the state dissolves over time. We have had the privilege of working with some patients for ten, twenty, and even thirty years, and have seen remarkable, lasting transformations.

PART I

Prevalence and Conventional Treatment of Depression, Anxiety and Bipolar Disorder

1 A Society of Mental and Emotional Imbalance

An Epidemic of Depression

Happiness is apparently not nearly as popular a topic as depression. "Compared with misery, happiness is relatively unexplored terrain for social scientists. Between 1967 and 1994, 46,380 articles indexed in *Psychological Abstracts* mentioned depression, 36,851 mention anxiety, and 5,099 articles mentioned anger. Only 2,389 articles spoke of happiness, 2,340 life satisfaction, and 405 joy." (Myers, p. 40) In 2000, however, was the inauguration of The Journal of Happiness Studies, a Dutch journal, which at least provides a place to publish serious research on happiness.

Depression is epidemic. According to the National Institute of Mental Health (NIMH), 6.7% of Americans are depressed at any one time, and 30.4% of those are considered severely depressed. Over a lifetime, 16.5% of people will be considered depressed. Women are 70% more likely than men to experience depression in their lifetime. Surprisingly, only 5% of those over 50 are depressed, compared with 9% of young adults 18-25. (NIMH "Major Depressive Disorder in Adults").

Chances are if you're not taking antidepressants, someone else you know is. There is a higher incidence of depression in younger people, blacks, those who are poorer, and in those who are separated or divorced rather than married or never married. (Blazer, p. 984-85) The number of office visits during which a psychiatric medication was prescribed increased from approximately 33 million in 1985 to 46 million in 1993 and 1994. Visits for depression increased from 11 million to over 20 million during the same decade while prescriptions of tranquilizers fell from 52% to 33% of psychotropic drugs due to the fact that doctors are favoring antidepressants. (Pincus, p. 529-30) "Given the number of people taking antidepressants, you may wonder if it is genuinely possible to be happy without a pill of some kind or other."

So did psychiatrist John Ratey of Harvard Medical School and Catherine Johnson of the National Alliance for Autism Research. In *Shadow Syndromes*, the authors argue that all sorts of quirky behaviors are actually mild mental illness. "The athletic megastar who is cool as ice in the championship game but explodes at a bar is not just a spoiled brat; he is beset by intermittent rage disorder. Men who are unable to talk about their feelings suffer from an 'unrecognized adult form of attention deficit disorder'. The deadbeat dad, who dotes on his children when they visit but who can't seem to remember to send the child-support checks has mild 'environmental dependency syndrome'. Whether it be a pre-anorexic teenage girl or a six-year-old with separation anxiety, Ratey and Johnson believe that drugs, most commonly antidepressants, are in order." (Begley, p. 52)

What Causes Depression?

It has been widely accepted for years that certain mental illnesses such as schizophrenia or bipolar disorder (manic depression) run in families. We have often observed family trends in patients with a variety of mental and emotional problems including depression, anxiety, bipolar disorder, obsessive compulsive disorder, attention deficit hyperactivity disorder, pathologic anger and violence, and drug addiction. It has long been argued whether these familial tendencies represent an actual genetic pre-disposition which is passed on from generation to generation or rather results from the environmental exposure of having grown up in a dysfunctional family.

Genetic researchers are investigating specific chromosomal correlations with a variety of mental and emotional states. In 1996, investigators at the National Cancer Institute identified a gene on chromosome 17 that contributes to becoming neurotic. (Begley, p. 54) Specific chromosomes have also been associated with obsessive-compulsive disorder (chromosome 22) and manic depression (chromosome 18). (Begley and

3

Ritter, p. 15) "The results of seven twin studies conducted in the United States, England, Germany, Norway and Denmark pegged the combined concordance rates for identical twins with affective disorders at 76% and found that 19% of the fraternal twins were concordant for affective [mood] disorders." (Papalos, p. 57)

It is no question that environmental factors can contribute to depression. The lack of nurturing, an atmosphere of neglect, drug and alcohol abuse, and sexual abuse can all turn an otherwise happy child to despair, low self-esteem and misery. Growing up in a household with a depressed family member, either parent, grandparent or sibling, can also instill feelings of gloom and guilt. The greatest preventive factor against depression, in our minds, is to grow up in a loving, supportive, communicative family. Rich or poor, it is this unconditional love which best instills the belief, "I am of value. I am loved. I am able to love. I am happy." Nevertheless, even well-loved and nurtured individuals with high self-esteem can still experience depression.

Another source of depression is situational. Difficult, challenging or tragic life events can result in a single episode of depression or recurrent pattern of sadness or despair. This pattern may result from the death or serious illness of a loved one, your own illness or chronic pain or fatigue, a career disappointment, lawsuit, bankruptcy, unhappy or dysfunctional relationships, abuse or neglect, family crisis or a spiritual dark night of the soul. Or from any number of physiologic conditions including pain, fatigue, thyroid imbalance, hormonal imbalances, sexual dysfunction, chemical sensitivities or addictions, poor eating habits or sleep disturbances. If you are healthy and have good coping skills, you will experience the sadness and pain, then move on with your life. If, however, you have not learned the adequate skills to deal with grief and depression, you may be mired in a quicksand of emptiness and hopelessness for months, years or life.

Certain pharmaceutical drugs, including some medications to lower blood pressure, cortisone, hormones such as estrogen and progesterone, and some drugs for cancer and Parkinson's disease can cause or aggravate depression. (Appleton, p. 161) The FDA, for example, issued a warning following reports of approximately a dozen patients who became severely depressed while taking the drug Accutane for acne. (*Newsweek*, "Is It the Pimples or the Pills?" p. 64) These people felt better when they discontinued the Accutane and their moods plummeted when they resumed taking it. Apparently manufacturer Hoffman-LaRoche had warned about depression in its Accutane literature for more than a decade. However, in 1998, the company advised doctors that "Accutane may cause depression, psychosis and, rarely... suicide". In this case, the cure was much worse than the disease.

It is important to research carefully the side effects of any medication that you take. Otherwise you may find yourself in a revolving door taking more and more medications to deal with the side effects of the ones you are already taking. This is particularly true with elderly people who may be taking even ten or more different prescription drugs.

The Serotonin Connection

The cause of depression which has most caught the attention of scientists in recent years is an imbalance of neurotransmitters, especially of serotonin. Researchers estimate the number of different neurotransmitters in the brain to be as many as 500. (Lemonick, p. 80) These chemicals, including serotonin, dopamine, norepinephrine and the hundreds of other known neurotransmitters as well as those yet undiscovered, are stored in tiny sacs located at nerve endings. From a neurological point of view, it is through these neurotransmitters that we are able to communicate with the outside world. (Lemonick, p. 76)

"The entire history of serotonin and of drugs that affect it has been largely a process of trial and error marked by chance discoveries, surprise connections and unanticipated therapeutic effects. The chemical was not even first discovered in the brain. It was stumbled onto in the late 1940's by U.S. and Italian researchers, working independently, in blood platelets and in the intestines, respectively." (Lemonick, p. 78). "Though serotonin has been known to researchers for nearly a half-century, only in recent years have neuroscientists begun to understand how important this one substance is to the functioning of the human psyche. Serotonin, or the lack of it, has been implicated not only in depression, uncontrollable appetite and obsessive-compulsive disorder, but also in autism, bulimia, social phobias, premenstrual syndrome, anxiety and panic, migraines, schizophrenia and even extreme violence." (Lemonick, p. 75) Researchers have also recently discovered that specially bred mice lacking a gene involved in the brain's response to serotonin were more motivated to take cocaine than normal mice (Allen, p. A9). If these findings pan out, drugs which regulate levels of serotonin may become useful in the prevention and treatment of drug addiction and prevention.

Researchers of the serotonin phenomenon have even found a mechanism to explain why women are more prone to depression than men. A recent study at McGill University, in which researchers measured serotonin secreted in the brains of eight healthy men and seven healthy women found that the men produced 52% more of the neurotransmitter than the women. (Nishizawa, p. 5308)

Yet, in spite of much study and impressive breakthroughs, researchers are only beginning to understand the chemical's complex role in the functioning of the body and brain. So far, the tools used to manipulate serotonin in the human brain are more like pharmacological machetes than they are like scalpels — crudely effective but capable of doing plenty of collateral damage. (Lemonick, p. 76) The drugs developed to enhance serotonin levels, the selective serotonin reuptake inhibitors (Prozac, Zoloft, Paxil, Effexor, Luvox and others), are effective clinically for a wide range of mental and emotional problems but their mechanism is not entirely understood. "At first it was thought that by blocking their re-uptake, the level of available serotonin was raised, but now it is known that the receptors are altered by becoming less sensitive." (Appleton, p. 54)

While researchers are hasty to jump on the serotonin bandwagon, fueled by the tremendous boom in serotonin-regulating pharmaceutical drugs, not everyone believes that neurotransmitters are the ultimate cause and cure of depression. Candice Pert, renowned as one of the original serotonin investigators, echoes a word of caution lest we jump too far too fast. "I am alarmed at the monster that Johns Hopkins neuroscientist Solomon Snyder and I created when we discovered the simple binding assay for drug receptors 25 years ago. Prozac and other antidepressant serotonin-receptor-active compounds may also cause cardiovascular problems in some susceptible people after long-term use, which has become common practice despite the lack of safety studies. The public is being misinformed about the precision of these selective serotonin-uptake inhibitors when the medical profession oversimplifies their action in the brain and ignores the body as if it exists merely to carry the head around! In short, these molecules of emotion regulate every aspect of our physiology. A new paradigm has evolved, with implications that life-style changes such as diet and exercise can offer profound, safe and natural mood elevation." (Pert, p. 8) Yet until another mechanism is suggested, the assumption that serotonin imbalance is the key determining factor in moods is the prevailing wisdom among scientists.

What Makes People Happy?

One common denominator among those who live long lives is a sense of mission or reason for their existence. Busy, service-oriented people have considerably less time to be depressed and to worry about themselves. The more you try to help others, the smaller you own problems, no matter how serious, will appear. "Apart from establishing an exercise program and improving diet, light, and sleep, the single most critical improvement anyone can make in brain function and in character, is to find a mission in life... an impassioned commitment to an activity pushes brain function in the direction of health, sanity and well-being." (Ratey and Johnson,

7

p. F2) If more people had deeply satisfying work, relationships, spiritual lives and a genuine sense of purpose, we can guarantee that the incidence of depression and need for antidepressants would be much diminished.

When researchers surveyed Americans to find out what made them happy, they found that contentment was not dependent on age, race, gender or wealth. In fact the 100 wealthiest Americans, according to Forbes Magazine, rated themselves as only slightly happier than the average American. The studies revealed that four traits consistently characterize happy people: they like themselves as people, feel as if they have personal control over their lives, are optimistic, and they are extroverted. Religiously active people also reported greater happiness. (Myers, p. 43)

How Effective Are Antidepressants?

Pick up a popular magazine such as *Newsweek*, look for a dark rain cloud and you will find a message from the Lilly pharmaceutical company. Beneath the grey, stormy cloud against a pitch-black background: "Prozac isn't a 'happy pill'. It's not a tranquilizer. It won't take away your personality. Depression can do that, but Prozac can't." Turn the page and a sun glows radiantly as it emerges from a perfectly blue sky assuring you that "Prozac can help... Prozac has been prescribed for more than 17 million Americans. Chances are someone you know is feeling sunny again because of it." Prozac has been one of the most in-demand and widely-prescribed drugs, with prescriptions in 1997 topping 22.8 million (Parade, p. 16) and annual sales of over one billion dollars (Breggin, p. 3).

Just who has gone from gloom to glee thanks to this phenomenally popular antidepressant? "These people range from children to adolescents to the elderly. Name any randomly chosen group of successful people in society, business, politics or the arts, and it is likely that 20% to 30% are either taking or have taken Prozac at some point over the last several years." (Fieve, p. 11)

If our nation has jumped on the Prozac bandwagon, it must be phenomenally effective. Yet a leading psychiatrist, Dr. Ronald Fieve, one of the foremost experts on the drug, cautions us that a mere 10% of those who do respond to Prozac show an extraordinary reaction while the other 90% of the patients do not undergo anything even vaguely like a transformation. "They simply come out of their depression." (Fieve, p. 3) Dr. Fieve continues, "In my private practice, I have seen a few patients utterly changed by Prozac, lifted from the deepest despair into an even-tempered, confident optimism. Their lives improved so suddenly and dramatically that they seemed to have new personalities. More often, however, the changes are less spectacular."

Anxiety

About 40 million Americas age 18 years old or over (about 18% of the population) suffer from anxiety disorders. (NIMH, "Anxiety Disorders") When we talk about anxiety, we include generalized anxiety disorder, panic disorder, agoraphobia, specific phobias, obsessive-compulsive disorder, social phobia, acute stress disorder and post-traumatic stress disorder. Anxiety disorders may accompany physical illnesses, other mental illnesses, or alcohol or substance abuse. Anxiety about health may lead to reading and researching obsessively about various health problems, and to convincing oneself that he suffers from them.

Generalized Anxiety Disorder refers to those individuals whose excessive worry about everyday issues and problems becomes chronic. Their concerns are persistent and overwhelming, even though they may be unwarranted and their life may, to the outside observer, be going quite smoothly without need for inordinate concern. They may be preoccupied with business of financial difficulties, family problems, work-related issues, health or anything else that disturbs them. Symptoms include sleep disturbance, inability to relax, difficulty concentrating and distractibility. Accompanying physical symptoms may be headaches, fatigue, sweating, nausea, lightheadedness, frequent urination, perspiration, restlessness or muscle tension.

Panic attacks are characterized by sudden terror along with a constellation of other symptoms which may include heart palpitations, perspiration, shortness of breath, a feeling of gasping, choking or smothering, chest pain, nausea, lightheadedness or dizziness, tingling and chills. They typically last only ten to fifteen minutes, but can be quite limiting, even debilitating. People often experience a strong desire to escape, exhibit avoidance behavior and may seek help from an emergency room for fear of having a heart attack. Panic disorder is twice as prevalent in women as in men. (Yonkers, K.A., et al., *Am J Psychiatry* 155:596-602, May 1998) Panic attacks may result in avoidance not only of a particular place or situation, but inability to engage in one's livelihood, to utilize modes of travel, and, in the case of agoraphobia, to leave the house. Requisite activities of normal, everyday living, such as driving, grocery shopping or going to work may become insurmountable and impossible, resulting in a state of incapacitation and social isolation.

About estimated 19.2 million adult Americans (8% of the population) suffer from one or more specific phobias, typically beginning in childhood (Kessler R.C., et al., p. 617-27) There is often evidence of phobia in other family members. These phobias generate intense, irrational fear and dread, often of activities or situations that, in reality, pose little or no actual threat or danger. Common phobias are of flying, elevators, bridges, tunnels, highways, water, injuries regarding blood and vomiting. Even when the intensity of the phobia is substantially diminished, there may remain a fear that the fear itself will return.

People with obsessive-compulsive disorder (OCD) experience a pattern of persistent, worrisome thoughts and use compulsive rituals to control the anxiety that results. Individuals who are germ-phobic may feel a need to wash their hands again and again or to shower repeatedly. Those who fear robbery, physical assault or danger to their homes may need to check over and over to make sure doors are locked, burners are turned off, and that they are not being followed. In some cases, the person may feel the need to follow a particular ritualized sequence, to count obsessively, or to do virtually any routine activity of life in a prescribed manner. OCD affects about 2.2 million American adults (ibid, p. 617-27), often running in families.

Social Anxiety Disorder (social phobia) is one that we treat commonly in our practice. It involves extreme self-consciousness about meeting new people, interacting with others in social settings or, especially, when they are called upon to speak or perform publicly. These individuals may feel okay in one-to-one encounters. However, we once treated a remarkably competent investment banker who, despite his years of expertise and experience, was overcome with anxiety, to the point of stuttering, even with his clients one-on-one. Such anxiety may arise from a humiliating experience in a classroom as a child or adolescent, or because of excessive, often unjustified, criticism from parents or teachers. It can also occur from a dysfunctional family situation of abuse, neglect or violence, where a feeling of safety and stability was lacking. The symptoms of social anxiety are similar to those of panic attacks: blushing, perspiration, trembling, nausea, stuttering or, in extreme cases, inability to speak or even fainting. One of our most articulate patients, highly skilled and respected in his field, still takes a homeopathic medicine for performance anxiety whenever he needs to address a large group. It is quite effective.

Post-traumatic stress disorder (PTSD) affects 7.7 million adults (Kessler R.C., et al., p. 617-27) and can be triggered in childhood or adolescence as well. It first came to light as a means of explaining the residual psychiatric disorders in soldiers after returning from war. However, any traumatic incident, whether child abuse, sexual abuse, rape, torture, riots, bombings, automobile accidents, natural disasters or near-death experiences may result in PTSD. It can occur either in the individual suffering the traumatic event or someone who witnessed it. Typical symptoms of PTSD are nightmares, flashbacks, insomnia, emotional detachment, startling, depression, loss of interest in life, aggressiveness, inability to give or receive affection or enjoy intimate relationships and substance abuse. There have also been correlations with borderline personality disorder or mutiple personality disorder.

Bipolar Disorder

Bipolar disorder is characterized by periodic, cyclic, dramatic mood swings. It is a complex illness and varies greatly from one individual to another. According to statistics from the National Institutes of Mental Health, it affects 2.6% of the adult population and up to 3% of adolescents. (Kessler R.C., et al., p. 617-27)

"Prevalence of child-onset bipolar disorder is not well established due to debate about the appropriate definition of boundaries of diagnosis among preadolescents." (NIMH, July 29, 2010) The ongoing debate regarding childhood bipolar disorder has been tainted by allegations of impropriety in the research conducted by Dr. Charles Biederman and associates at Harvard University in conjunction with pharmaceutical companies, resulting in a disproportional increase in the diagnosis of pediatric bipolar disorder and the use of highly profitable atypical antipsychotic medications to treat it. (See Chapter 3).

Symptoms of the manic phase of adult bipolar disorder include excessive happiness, irritability, excitement, euphoria, restlessness, agitation, erratic behavior and conversation, decreased need for sleep, racing thoughts, rapid, pressured speech, increased energy and physical activity, a tendency to make unrealistic, unattainable plans, a heightened libido, inconsistency in attendance at work or school, spending sprees, faulty financial decisions and, in some cases, psychotic thinking. The individual may exhibit careless or dangerous use of drugs or alcohol. The phase of depression may include sadness, hopelessness, anxiety, irritability, difficulty concentrating, diminished energy, uncontrollable crying, fluctuating appetite, increased need for sleep, difficulty making decisions and suicidal thoughts or behavior. Moods may vary seasonally.

Bipolar individuals may be brilliant, talented, creative, artistic and highly successful in their careers. They tend to be intense in whatever they do. Engaging, gregarious, charismatic and great company when their moods are stable, people with bipolar disorder may become boisterous, loquacious, pushy and overall too much to handle for those around them. Sadly, those suffering from bi-polar disorder tend to lose friendships, families and fortunes during their manic episodes and to burn their bridges so that no one is left to support them through their ups and downs. It is extremely important to pay attention to suicidal ideation in a patient with bipolar disorder, during manic or depressive episodes, because 10% to 15% of people with bipolar disorder commit suicide. (*Web MD*) In children and adolescents, diagnosis is often based on explosive temper, rapid mood shifts, aggressive behavior and erratic sleep patterns. Many children receive this diagnosis based primarily on behavior, without any clear-cut depression or mania.

2 Antidepressants, Anti-Anxiety Medications, Antipsychotics and Mood Stabilizers

A Pill for Every Ill

Physicians have been treating depression, anxiety, OCD and bipolar disorder with a range of medications with varying levels of success for over 50 years. Psychiatry has gone though various phases in treatment, with new generation medications replacing older ones as treatment protocols changed and patents on older drugs ran out, making them less profitable.

Tricyclic antidepressants, e.g. Tryptizol (amitriptyline), Anafranil (clomipramine), Tofranil (imipramine), and MAO (monoamine oxidase) inhibitors, e.g. Parnate (tranylcypromine), Nardil (phenelzine), though often neglected today, were the backbone of depression treatment for more than a generation. MAO inhibitors were most often used only when other antidepressants were ineffective, because of their many drug and food interactions, which could cause serious hypertensive crisis or serotonin syndrome. Prozac (fluoxetine), which came to market in 1987, and the other SSRIs (selective serotonin reuptake inhibitors), such as Zoloft (sertraline) and Paxil (paroxetine), were the new generation in the late 80s and early 90s.

The benzodiazepines, e.g. Valium (diazepam), Librium (chlordiazepoxide), Xanax (alprazolam) and Ativan (lorazepam), were used for decades for both acute and chronic anxiety, until chronic use was found to cause dependance with severe withdrawal symptoms for many patients. (Longo and Johnson, p. 2121-30). Now the SSRIs, including Zoloft, Lexapro, Paxil and Luvox, and the newer SSNRIs (selective serotonin norepinephrine reuptake inhibitors), such as Effexor (venlafaxine), Cymbalta (duloxetene) and Pristiq (desvenlafaxine), have largely replaced them for treating chronic anxiety states. The benzodiazepines, however, are still commonly used for acute or severe, but short-term anxiety states where dependance is not an issue.

For bipolar disorder, lithium carbonate has been the workhorse of treatment for mania alternating with depression since 1970. Anticonvulsant/mood stabilizers, e.g. Depakote (valproic acid), Lamictal (lamotrigene), Tegretol (carbamazapine), and atypical antipsychotics, such as Risperdal (risperidone), Abilify (aripriprazole), Geodon (ziprasidone) and Seroquel (quetiapine), are increasingly being used with or without lithium in bipolar patients. The atypical antipsychotics have had the most dramatic rise in prescriptions, especially in children with or without bipolar disorder and the elderly, especially nursing home patients with dementia. (Harris, p. A20, Motsinger, et al., p. 2335-41). This is despite their clear side effects of weight gain and a substantial link to increased risk of diabetes.

SSRIs: Getting a Rise Out of Serotonin

The antidepressant renaissance began in 1987 with the introduction of Prozac (fluoxetine). A media phenomenon, the drug aroused more public interest than any other before or since, except perhaps Viagra, the impotency wonder drug. Sensationalized on numerous television talk shows and major magazine covers, Prozac appeared to be a panacea for many or all of those suffering from depression. It is still quite popular, especially since 2001 in generic versions, with over 24.3 million prescriptions in 2009. (*drugtopics.com*, 2010)

Prozac was developed specifically for the treatment of depression, designed to act only on the serotonin system. Its strongest selling point is its minimal side effects compared to its predecessors, the older families of tri-cyclic antidepressants and MAO inhibitors. Although Prozac's initial indications were only for depression, it is now widely used for a number of other conditions including obsessive-compulsive disorder, bulimia, panic disorder and social phobias in adults and children.

Soon after Prozac was introduced, other SSRIs came to market in the 90s and early 2000s including Paxil (paroxetine), Luvox (fluvoxamine), Zoloft (sertraline), Celexa (citalopram) and

15

Lexapro (escitalopram). What ties these drugs together is the principle of maintaining higher levels of serotonin, a neurotransmitter in the brain, by slowing its reuptake (re-absorption) at the synapses between the nerve cells. The higher concentration of serotonin at the synapse enhances nerve conduction and stimulation. In practical terms, when serotonin levels are higher, the nerves fire more often, and patients with depression, anxiety, OCD and other conditions tend to improve.

Happy as a Clam

"How do you get a clam in the mood? Take it to a clam bar? Won't work — white wine goes with clams, but only so far. And, let's face it, big mussels are a turnoff. So what's left? Well, you might try Prozac. It works for Peter Fong." ("Clam Dunk", *People*, p. 79).

The most surprising application of Prozac that we have come across is to improve on Mother Nature by helping clams to spawn. Apparently, according to biologist Peter Fong of Gettysburg College, the drug gets them in a spawning mood. (Reuters, p. 19) Dr. Fong discovered that just one drop of Prozac makes clams act like rabbits. In just one hour each happy clam produces ten little baby clams. ("Clam Dunk", *People*, p. 79) His research suggests that Prozac effects mollusks in the same way as humans by increasing the secretion of serotonin. Biologists have long known that serotonin induces spawning behavior in clams and mussels but Prozac may increase effectiveness and lower costs for aquatic farmers. This may even give rise to a new profession: mollusk psychiatry. (Reuters, p. 19) Research has not been done on humans, lest you may be tempted to consider Prozac as an aphrodisiac.

118 Million Prescriptions

Apparently trying to make people as happy as the clams, American physicians wrote 118 million prescriptions for antidepressants in 2004, according to a study by the Centers for Disease Control and Prevention. (*CNN health.com*)

All of the antidepressants, new and old, are equally effective for major depression, however the newer drugs have significant advantages regarding safety and side effects. The growing awareness of serotonin's important role in mood and emotion has been paralleled, and sometimes driven by, a boom in drugs that target serotonin.

A 2009 meta-analysis of 117 studies comparing the twelve most popular new generation antidepressants (SSRIs and SSNRIs) concluded that for parameters of cost, efficacy and acceptability for patients, Zoloft and Lexapro, the patent-extending version of Celexa, ranked the highest. Also, Zoloft edged out Lexapro in the analysis by being the less costly of the two. These two drugs were followed in the popularity ratings by Prozac, Paxil, Cymbalta and Luvox. (Cipriani, et al., p. 746-58)

Drugs such as these have changed many lives for the better, but they also have their downsides as well. It's best to be fully informed before choosing how you want to treat your depression, anxiety or other mental and emotional issues, and whether you would like to consider a complementary or alternative medicine such as homeo-pathy as the means of changing your life and health for the better.

3 Designer Drugs

The Price You May Pay

As you can see by perusing the *Physician's Desk Reference* (www.pdr.net), the reference guide to prescription medications, all drugs have side effects, some more dangerous or annoying than others. Although conventional medicine can be of great benefit for a variety of conditions, it is your responsibility to inform yourself about the side effects, contraindications and possible drug interactions of the medication you are taking. Otherwise, the price you pay may be more than just the cost of the drug.

For example, Zoloft can trigger anxiety, agitation, headache, nausea and diarrhea. Zoloft, Prozac and many other SSRIs may cause sexual dysfunction. Paxil is known to sedate and to cause dry mouth and constipation. Luvox can cause increased fatigue and tremors. All these symptoms are annoying to be sure, yet they are a price that many depressed patients have been willing to pay to reduce their symptoms and suffering.

One psychiatrist suggested that a friend of ours named Stephen try Prozac. When Stephen inquired about the well-known decrease in libido in Prozac-users, the doctor replied, "Most people who are depressed don't care about sex anyway." Stephen's reply: "No thanks. I do care about sex."

Monkeying with the chemistry of the human mind can trigger problems much more serious than a dull sex life. In 1997, just 1½ years after it approved Redux (dexfenfluramine), an SSRI, for treatment of obesity, the FDA issued a warning advising patients to stop taking it and its close chemical cousin fenfluramine. The combination of fenfluramine and phentarmine (fen-phen) could potentially cause serious, even fatal cardiac weakness due to disease of the mitral or aortic valves. (Lemonick, p. 75-6).

Please see the sidebar below, in which the various SSRIs are differentiated by the conditions they best treat and by side effect profiles. Although the SSRIs are quite similar in their indications and side effect profiles, there can be subtle differences that make one more suitable than another on an individual basis.

SSRIs	Indications	Prominent Side Effects
All	Major Depressive Disorder Obsessive-Compulsive Disorder (OCD) Panic Disorder Social Anxiety Disorder Premenstrual Dysphoric Disorder (PMDD) or Pre-Menstrual Syndrome (PMS) Post-Traumatic Stress Disorder (PTSD)	Low libido Orgasm problems Impotence Ejaculation problems Increased risk of suicide in children and young adults Agitation Apathy Anxiety Panic Nervousness Hostility or aggression Elation alternating with depression Dry mouth Headache Nausea Diarrhea Constipation Indigestion Appetite changes Shaking (tremors) Restlessness Dizziness Weight gain Drowsiness Insomnia Yawning

SSRIs	Indications	Prominent Side Effects
		Fatigue Weakness Allergic reactions Rash, hives Increased sweating Dilated pupils Weight gain or loss Photosensitivity (sunburn) Paresthesia
Zoloft (sertraline)	Major Depressive Disorder Obsessive-Compulsive Disorder (OCD) Panic Disorder Social Anxiety Disorder Premenstrual Dysphoric Disorder (PMDD) or Pre-Menstrual Syndrome (PMS) Post-Traumatic Stress Disorder (PTSD)	Ejaculation failure Decreased libido Dry mouth Increased sweating Sleepiness Dizziness Headache Tremor Diarrhea Indigestion Nausea Fatigue Insomnia Restlessness
Lexapro (escitalo-pram)	Major Depressive Disorder Generalized Anxiety Disorder	Ejaculation delay Decreased libido Lack of orgasm Nausea Diarrhea Insomnia Sleepiness Dry mouth

SSRIs	Indications	Prominent Side Effects
		Fatigue Constricted pupils Dizziness Restlessness
Prozac (fluox- etine)	Major Depressive Disorder Obsessive- Compulsive Disorder (OCD) Panic Disorder Bulimia Nervosa Post-Traumatic Stress Disorder (PTSD)	Headache Weakness Nausea Diarrhea Anorexia Dry mouth Indigestion Insomnia Nervousness Sleepiness Dizziness Tremor Sweating
Paxil (parox- etene)	Major Depressive Disorder Obsessive- Compulsive Disorder (OCD) Generalized Anxiety Disorder Panic Disorder Social Anxiety Disorder	Nausea Sleepiness Weakness Weight gain Insomnia Constipation Tremor Suicidal risk in children and adults Withdrawal syndrome Low libido Orgasm problems Mania Birth defects

Luvox (fluoxetine)	Major Depressive Disorder Obsessive Compulsive Disorder Generalized Anxiety Disorder Panic Disorder Social Phobia Post-Traumatic Stress Disorder (PTSD)	Nausea Weakness Dyspepsia Sleepiness Anorexia Dental problems Loss of appetite Nervousness Tremor Dizziness Sweating Ejaculation problems Orgasm problems Respiratory infections
Celexa (citalopram)	Major Depressive Disorder Off-Label Uses: ADHD Obsessive-Compulsive Disorder (OCD) Body Dysmorphic Disorder (BDD) Premenstrual Dysphoric Disorder (PMDD)	Dry mouth Orgasm problems Ejaculation problems Drowsiness Insomnia Nausea Sweating Tremor Diarrhea Fatigue Anxiety Mood swings

Not Necessarily a Quick Fix

People who are quite depressed are often, with good reason, looking for a rapid or immediate answer. Unfortunately, regardless of which therapy you use, this may not be possible. Although the response rate [to SSRI's] in severe depression is adequate, the cure rate is low and slow for the SSRI's and "... they are not miracle drugs. Patients with severe depression must tolerate weeks and months of waiting before they truly feel better." (Appleton, p. 58)

Even experts in the field admit that antidepressants aren't the answer for everyone. "It has been estimated that 40% of those who have tried an antidepressant cannot tolerate the side effects or do not respond to the first drug with which they are treated. Of these, an additional 50% respond to a second antidepressant. This leaves 20% who fail to respond to the second drug. They are given one of several drugs in addition to the second antidepressant." (Fieve, p. 48-9)

The SSRI antidepressants are much better tolerated than their predecessors. However, according to Dr. William Appleton, a psychiatrist on the faculty of Harvard Medical School, "about 15 to 20% of people who take them cannot tolerate the abdominal distress or 'drugged' feeling, or other side effects, and must stop taking the medication. An equal number do not improve, so that the figure of about 40 or more % who fail to improve on their first antidepressant remains. This situation is not unique to psychiatry." (Appleton, p. 49)

"A study by A.C. Pande and M.E. Sayler (1993) of 3,183 outpatients in nineteen controlled studies of Prozac compared with a placebo or an older antidepressant found a remission rate in the severely depressed of only 27 to 29% on Prozac, 26% on a tri-cyclic antidepressant and 18% on a placebo. These results are far from spectacular and demonstrate the need for the physician to carefully follow severely depressed patients and not merely send them off with a Prozac prescription in the naive belief that they will all get better." (Appleton, p. 53)

What Is Meant by "Better"?

Some patients claim major improvement from antidepressants, however a fair number of patients report a partial improvement and still take little or no pleasure in life. (Appleton, p. 50) Perhaps 90% of the patients who respond to Prozac will not experience dramatic results. "They do not undergo anything even vaguely like a transformation. They simply come out of their depression... Perhaps 10% of those who do respond to Prozac show an extraordinary reaction." (Fieve, p. 3)

According to a 2010 meta-analysis of the effectiveness of antidepressants, "The magnitude of benefit of antidepressant medication compared with placebo increases with severity of depression symptoms and may be minimal or nonexistent, on average, in patients with mild or moderate symptoms. For patients with very severe depression, the benefit of medications over placebo is substantial." (Fournier et. al, p. 47-53)

Another question is how long the individual continues to feel better from a drug such as Prozac as opposed to the uplifting effect diminishing over time or to that person experiencing side effects down the road. In order for the FDA (Food and Drug Administration) to introduce a new antidepressant in the marketplace, it must be judged safe and effective. However, this requires a four to six week controlled clinical trial including about 2,500 patients. In reality only several hundred of these patients are observed for more than a few months. Many psycho-pharmacologists have recommended longer trials both to assure that long term, not just short term, statistical improvement occurs and to discover long term side effects. (Appleton, p. 34-5)

How much better can a depressed person expect to feel? In most cases, in our clinical experience with homeopathic medicine, considerably better. Unfortunately there are few clinical trials on homeopathic treatment of depression. A new double-blind study comparing individualized homeopathic treatment with 20 mg of daily Prozac, found comparably successful results with the two approaches in 91 randomly assigned outpatients with moderate to severe depression. Patients in the Prozac group, however, had more side effects and some dropped out of the study for this reason. (Adler, et al., p. 1-8) We look forward to the day when enough research has been done that we can definitely and accurately compare the results of SSRIs and homeopathy in the treatment of depression. In our experience, a significant portion of depressed patients feel significantly happier and more energetic, and some have a life-transforming response, as you can see for yourselves as you read the case histories in this book.

What About Withdrawal from Antidepressants?

If you decide to discontinue taking antidepressants while under homeopathic treatment, we recommend that you do so under the guidance of your prescribing physician. You may experience flu-like symptoms when you try to come off of your SSRI's and feel generally bad. This does not necessarily mean that you must continue taking your antidepressants; you may simply need to be weaned off of them more gradually. Although some people do have difficulty in stopping Prozac, it is generally easier to discontinue than many other drugs due to its long action. Other antidepressants, such as Paxil, Zoloft and Effexor, can be much more difficult to discontinue. Withdrawal symptoms include continuation of the common side effects experienced while using the drugs (see SSRI side bar above), with emphasis on "brain zaps", a kind of variable electric shock sensation, and various type of sexual dysfunction (see sidebar above).

Antidepressants, Mood Stabilizers and Atypical Antipsychotics for Kids

We have treated over 3000 children for attention deficit hyperactivity disorder and other behavioral and learning problems. Initially we were surprised to hear that, in addition to Ritalin or other stimulant medications, Prozac or other SSRIs were part of the daily treatment regimen of some of these kids. Some tolerate the drugs well; others do not.

In a recent editorial in the Townsend Letter for Doctors and Patients, noted complementary and alternative medical doctor Alan Gaby spoke about the over-medication of children in today's society. "More than 25% of American children and teenagers are being medicated. Among children aged 9 years or younger, there are 45 million prescriptions or refills dispensed each year for asthma medications, 7 million prescriptions or refills each year for attention deficit/hyperactivity disorder (ADHD) drugs, 1 million for antidepressants, 1.4 million for antipsychotic drugs, 1.8 million for antihypertensive medications, 30,000 for type 2 diabetes, and 11,000 for statin drugs."

(Gaby, p. 107) He felt that the quantity of children being medicated was disturbing and that some of the drugs involved were studied primarily or exclusively for adults, resulting in little or no information on proper dosing or attention to safety or efficacy in children.

The increased use of medication in the young indicated that their level of health was clearly declining, with more serious health problems occurring at more tender ages.

Another, earlier warning was issued by Mary Crowley, in a *Newsweek* article in 1997. "A generation after depressed adults started listening to Prozac, a generation of children is tuning in. None of the half-dozen drugs in Prozac's class, the so-called selective serotonin reuptake inhibitors, has been fully tested in children. But because the drugs are FDA-approved for use in adults, doctors can legally prescribe them to kids as well. The new users span every sector of society, from Manhattan's most elite schools to Atlanta's poorest ones, and their numbers are exploding." (Crowley, p. 73)

Children age 6 to 18 received 735,000 SSRI prescriptions in 1996, an increase of 80% in just two years. Researchers at the University of Texas Southwestern Medical Center gave Prozac or a placebo to 96 depressed children and adolescents: mood ratings improved after eight weeks in 56% of the Prozac-treated kids versus a third on placebo. This is about the same effectiveness as with adults. But the study also turned up a worrisome potential side effect not seen in adults: 6% of the treated children became manic. (Crowley, p. 74)

Between 1996 and 2005, use of antidepressants doubled for both children and adults from 5% to over 10% of the population in the U.S., approximately 27 million people. Those who received antidepressant treatment were also more likely to be prescribed antipsychotic medicines and less likely to receive psychotherapy. (Olfson, M, and Marcus, S, p. 848-56)

Preventing or Promoting Suicide in Children: A Controversy over SSRI Use

In 2004, the FDA issued a black box warning for all antidepressants, revised in 2007 and excerpted below:

Suicidality and Antidepressant Drugs

Antidepressants increased the risk compared to placebo of suicidal thinking and behavior (suicidality) in children, adolescents and young adults in short-term studies of major depressive disorder (MDD) and other psychiatric disorders.

Anyone considering the use of [Insert established name] or any other antidepressant in a child, adolescent or young adult must balance this risk with the clinical need. Short-term studies did not show an increase in the risk of suicidality with antidepressants compared to placebo in adults beyond age 24; there was a reduction in risk with antidepressants compared to placebo in adults aged 65 and older. Depression and certain other psychiatric disorders are themselves associated with increases in the risk of suicide. Patients of all ages who are started on antidepressant therapy should be monitored appropriately and observed closely for clinical worsening, suicidality or unusual changes in behavior. Families and caregivers should be advised of the need for close observation and communication with the prescriber. [Insert Drug Name] is not approved for use in pediatric patients. [The previous sentence would be replaced with the sentence, below, for the following drugs: Prozac: Prozac is approved for use in pediatric patients with MDD and obsessive compulsive disorder (OCD). Zoloft: Zoloft is not approved for use in pediatric patients except for patients with obsessive compulsive disorder (OCD). Fluvoxamine: Fluvoxamine is not approved for use in pediatric patients except for patients with obsessive compulsive disorder (OCD).

Since the above warning was issued, there has been controversy about whether the risk of prescribing antidepressants for suicidal depressed children, adolescents and young adults up to age 24 is worse than the risk of failing to treat depressed young people who may otherwise go on to attempt or commit suicide. It appears that the suicide risk for young people is greatest in the first one to two months of antidepressant treatment and after that becomes less. The warning has dramatically decreased the use of SSRIs in young people, but the suicide rate as of 2007 had not increased over 2006. (Xu J, et al.)

A 2006 study of children under 14 on SSRIs indicated that higher prescription rates were associated with fewer actual suicides, but cautioned that there was not necessarily a causal relationship. (Gibbons, et al., p. 1356-63)

Until more extensive studies are completed on the long-term side-effects of antidepressants in children, we are very reticent about their use. Especially since we have found homeopathy can be extremely effective in treating a wide variety of mental and emotional problems in youngsters.

A Typical Prescription: Atypical Antipsychotics

More alarming has been the substantial rise in the rate of children diagnosed with Pediatric Bipolar Disorder and prescribed anti-seizure drugs such as Depakote (valproic acid) and Tegretol (carbamazapine) and the new generation of atypical antipsychotic medications including Risperdal (risperidone) introduced in 1993, Abilify (arapiprazole), Seroquel (quetiapine), Zyprexa (olanzapine) and Geodon (ziprazidone). These drugs are also prescribed for oppositional, aggressive or hyperactive children as well.

The major proponent of the new diagnosis and its related medications, Dr. Charles Biederman, and his associates, Dr. Thomas Spencer and Dr. Timothy Wilens, well known researchers in bipolar disorder and ADHD, were censured in July 2011 by Harvard University for accepting undisclosed payments amounting to more than a million dollars each from the pharmaceutical industry in connection with their research studies. (Convey)

This casts a cloud over the veracity of their research, which forms the basis for much of the increase in the use of antipsychotic medications for PBD and ADHD. These potential improprieties were brought to light in 2008 by Senator Charles E. Grassley, who accused them of receiving millions of dollars in unreported payments. (Harris, p. A20)

According to a 2008 article in the *N.Y. Times*, more than 389,000 U.S. children were being prescribed Risperdal in 2007, more than 240,000 under age ten. Many of them were treated for ADHD, which is off-label use of the drug. The side effects of Risperdal include substantial weight gain, metabolic problems and the risk of permanent symptoms of tardive dyskinesia, a movement disorder long associated with old and newer generations of antipsychotics. (Harris, p. A20)

In a 2011 report of inpatient use of antipsychotic medications in 3,851 patients, 44% of the patients were receiving antipsychotic medication for a variety of conditions, including psychosis and mood and anxiety, 94% receiving the newer generation of atypical antipsychotics. The study also indicated the use of atypical psychotics in children in outpatient settings quadrupled between 1997 and 2002, indicating the popularity of the new drugs. ("Examining Atypical Antipsychotic Use in Children", *Physician's Weekly*, 2011)

According to another recent article in the *N.Y. Times*, "The new generation of antipsychotic medications has also become the single biggest target of the False Claims Act, a federal law once largely aimed at fraud among military contractors. Every major company selling the drugs — Bristol-Myers Squibb, Eli Lilly, Pfizer, AstraZeneca and Johnson & Johnson — has either settled recent government cases for hundreds of millions of dollars or is currently under investigation for possible health care fraud." (Wilson, 2010)

The Dangers of Drug Interactions

The following types of drugs all interact with SSRIs and must be used with caution:

anticonvulsants	lithium	tri-cyclic antidepressants
antiarrhythmics	antipsychotics	beta-blockers
antihistamines	anticoagulants	antiulcer drugs
antianxiety drugs	phenothiazine	some over-the-counter cough or sleep medications containing alcohol

MAO inhibitors and trytophan must be avoided with the SSRIs. (Appleton, p. 83)

If you are taking any other prescription medication and are concerned about the possible interaction with an antidepressant, consult with any prescribing physician for further information.

There are also a number of pharmaceuticals that can cause or worsen depression. They include Inderal, Catapres, Aldomet and Reserpine for hypertension, cortisone, estrogen and progesterone, chemotherapeutic drugs such as vincristine and vinblastine, and Sinemat and amantadine for Parkinson's disease. (Appleton, p. 161)

4 A Matter of Personal Choice

Are Drugs the Answer for Me?

What Do People Say Who Have Taken Antidepressants?

Millions of people are taking antidepressants. It is not surprising that their experiences are vastly varied. Here are some comments about Prozac, the flagship of the SSRI antidepressants.

On the up side: "My personality has completely reversed. I was so sullen and antisocial before. Now I smile and I go out of my way to meet people and to make friends. I can concentrate again."

In the middle: "Happy I'm not. Never was. Never will be. But profoundly depressed, I'm not."

And on the negative side: "Even though at least three doctors had told me the Prozac was not causing my headaches, I decided to stop taking it... and the headaches went away! I spent a year of my life suffering from the worst headaches you can imagine and they were gone within two weeks of ending the Prozac." "[Prozac] left me (a 79-year-old mother and grandmother) in such a debilitated state, both mentally and physically. My daughter had to take care of everything for me. I lost my appetite and went from 167 pounds to 112 pounds. My daughter and I complained to the doctor, suggested that Prozac was weakening my system. But he insisted I continue taking Prozac. I refused so he refused to take care of me. I stopped and he stopped, but I'm the better for it... It has taken me almost a year and a half to recuperate."

Some derived benefit from Prozac but struggle with the dilemma of whether or not to take it for life. "It has been four and a half years since I stopped taking Prozac and lithium... I try very hard to live my life without medication. Sometimes I think it would be easier to just take it again, but my heart tells me no." Or "My doctor and I have now discussed the possibility that I may have to take Prozac for the rest of my life. If that is the case,

31

I have no problem with it. I hope to one day go off Prozac to see what happens, but I can assure you that if I have further depression, I will be back on it as soon as possible." (All comments in the last three paragraphs are from Elfenbein, p. 14-167)

Different people, different opinions. Hearing these personal experiences does, however, provide a reality check. A miracle for some, a curse for others. And, in some cases, a drug on which they are dependent for the rest of their lives. For them, no Prozac means no happiness. Effectiveness aside, side effects of the SSRIs still cause about 20% of those taking them to discontinue within six weeks and probably another 10% within the first year. (Appleton, p. 82)

What's Best for You?

Only you can decide what is the best course to follow. By all means, gather all the information you can. Read the latest books on all the various approaches to depression, surf the internet, talk to friends. The best choice is an informed choice. Here are a few guidelines to help decide what's right for you:

- Exactly how bad do you feel? Hopeless enough that you would seriously consider ending your life? If so, we recommend that you contact your local crisis team immediately. You may need hospitalization and are likely to need medication under the guidance of and psychotherapy with a professional skilled in working with suicidal patients.
- If you have been taking antidepressants with considerable to great success, are quite satisfied with them and feel no qualms about continuing them for the rest of your life, you have probably already found your answer.
- If you have mild to moderate depression, have tried antidepressants with little success or are disturbed by the side effects and are looking for a different approach, an alternative such as homeopathy might be just what you're seeking.

- If antidepressants work okay for you but you just can't see yourself taking them for the next year or for the rest of your life, we suggest you explore the other options.
- If you're happy with your antidepressants but someone else, a parent, family member or friend, tries to talk you out of taking them, listen to yourself, not to them.
- If you've tried other natural approaches to treat depression such as St. John's wort, nutritional supplements or other over the counter products and are not satisfied with the results, you may be an excellent candidate for homeopathy.
- Once you are clear about your decision, stick by it without any apologies. If you later realize it was not the right decision for you, it is fine to change your mind.

One of the best pieces of advice we have heard from a psychiatrist regarding the decision whether or not to take antidepressants is the following: "Who knows what miracle medication will come along next year, genetically engineered to root out the elusive depressive gene? Somehow I suspect humans do not work that way, and that our machine requires more than a drug. It requires love and useful activity of which we can be proud, and the identification of something worth living for. It takes more than Prozac to make a full life." (Appleton, p. 183) We couldn't agree more.

Don't Take Antidepressants, Wear Them!

For those of you who are hesitating to take Prozac or other medications to enounter depression, there's another option. "It's like a charm," says artist Colleen Wolstenholme of the silver jewelry she makes from castings of actual pills from Dexedrine to Zoloft, Xanax and Ativan. Dangling from the necks, ears and wrists of thousands, some people think that if they wear it, they won't have to take it. (*Newsweek*, Trend, 8) If it helps them feel better, more power to them. At least they don't have to worry about any side effects.

33

PART II

Homeopathy: An Effective Answer for Depression

5 What Is Homeopathy and How Does It Work?

Safe and Effective Natural Medicine with a Two-Hundred-Year Track Record

A Gentler Medicine

A little over two hundred years ago a dedicated and brilliant Geman physician, Samuel Hahnemann, became disillusioned with the medicine of his time which his colleagues called "heroic" and he called "barbaric". Crude treatments such as bloodletting, purging and the use of toxic substances including arsenic and mercury were commonplace. George Washington, in a futile effort to relieve a persistent fever, was one of the unfortunate men who died from bloodletting by his well-meaning but ineffective physicians.

Hahnemann was convinced not only that there must be safer, gentler and more effective methods of treatment, but that there must be consistent principles by which people became ill and healed. Through extensive experimentation and clinical trials, Hahnemann, with the help of his students and his colleagues, developed the principles and practice of homeopathic medicine. By the mid-1820's homeopathy had spread throughout Europe and to the United States. Homeopathic medical schools, hospitals and sanitariums flourished throughout the 19th century. In fact, by 1900 one out of every six physicians in this country practised homeo-pathy. Homeopathy continued to grow in popularity in Europe. However, due primarily to political reasons and to the increasing predominance of pharmaceutical drugs, nearly all of the homeopathic medical schools in the U.S. closed in the early part of this century. By the 1930's and 40's a small number of older homeopaths were still in practice but no further training was available. In the late 1970's homeopathy began to experience a resurgence in this country. This so-called renaissance has continued and the popularity of homeopathic medicine has grown tremendously, particularly over the past five years.

As You Ail, So You Heal

Homeopathy is a unique form of medicine with its own philosophy, medicines and methods of treatment. Although it is often confused with a variety of other forms of natural healing and alternative medicine, it is a medical art and science which stands by itself. The single principle on which homeopathy is fundamentally based is the *law of similars* or like cures like. This means that the same substance which causes a particular set of symptoms in a healthy person can relieve similar symptoms in a person who is ill. This is where the term homeopathy, meaning "similar suffering", originated.

For example, a person who is stung by a bee experiences swelling, redness, heat and burning or stinging pain of the local area. These symptoms can be relieved by a homeopathic medicine called *Apis mellifica* which is prepared from a honeybee. However *Apis* can be effective not only for bee stings, but for other conditions in which the same symptom picture is present. These include allergic reactions, inflammatory arthritis and bladder infections, especially when the main complaint is swelling.

Homeopaths often refer to conventional medicine as *allopathic* medicine. This comes from the Greek root *allo*, meaning "different". Modern medicine tends to use medicines which work against a particular condition or disease such as anti-biotics, anti-inflammatories, anti-fungals and anti-histamines. The goal of conventional medicine is to fight disease while homeopathy attempts to strengthen or balance the organism so that the person is no longer susceptible to illness.

The Unique Integration of Each Person

Integral to the philosophy of homeopathic medicine is to understand that each person is a whole. The hallmark of modern medicine is specialization. If you have a specific medical problem beyond the general scope of a family practice physician, you

37

will be sent to one or more specialists, each attending to one particular part of your body. You may see a rheumatologist for your arthritis, a podiatrist for bunions, an internist for gastritis and a cardiologist for hypertension. This is not unusual; in fact it is the norm. One doctor often does not know what the other is doing or which medicines you're taking. The result is often a long list of prescription medications with a potentially long list of side effects, especially when combined with one other.

There are many types of natural therapies that fall under the umbrella of *holistic* medicine. Yet, while the goal is said to be treating you as a whole person, the practitioners still prescribes different medicines or therapies for your digestive system, your adrenal glands or the nerves. From a homeopathic perspective, this is still treating the person piecemeal.

Homeopathy emphasizes the *totality of symptoms*. This means that every symptom you have must be taken in account in order to understand what about you needs to be healed. Each individual is an integrated, unique organism with a variety of characteristics and symptoms. As homeopaths, we do not believe it is possible to separate the head from feet or the mind from the body. We are like jigsaw puzzles with many intricate pieces of varying sizes and shapes. It is only when each and every piece is assembled that the picture of you as an individual is clearly recognizable.

Homeopathy not only takes into account each and every symptom, but treats them as well. If your chief complaint is anxiety but you also suffer from headaches, heartburn and joint pain, you should expect to notice an improvement in all of these areas. Since homeopathy is an integrated, whole person approach, all of you, rather than just your individual parts, will be stimulated to heal.

Individualized Medicines

Each person is one of a kind. No two people are the same in every way, even identical twins. Even if human beings, like sheep, are cloned, they will be genetically identical but different in other ways due to life experience and environment.

There are over two thousand homeopathic medicines and more are being introduced all the time. The task of the homeopath is to thoroughly understand the patient and the medicines and to make the best possible match. As you have just learned, every homeopathic medicine fits a specific set of symptoms. The more common medicines may fit thousands of symptoms, the more unusual ones at least a dozen. Each medicine has a pattern of symptoms as does each person. In *classical homeopathy*, the method taught by Hahnemann and the one that we, and many other homeopaths, espouse, only one single medicine is used at a time. If you go into a health food store, you can find homeopathic combination preparations containing a number of different medicines, but that is not the type of homeopathy that we practise or that is recommended in this book.

In first-aid conditions such as sprains or burns, which you can often treat yourself, the symptoms selected are fairly routinely based solely on that injury. Acute conditions such as colds, flu, diarrhea or sore throats are a bit more complicated. The homeopath takes into account each one of your symptoms that has changed since you became ill. In chronic conditions, however, such as depression, anxiety, asthma, ulcers, allergies or headaches, every aspect, symptom or characteristic that makes you different from everyone else must be taken into account.

This is why homeopathic practitioners spend such a long time with each patient. It takes a minimum of an hour and a half for an adult and an hour for a child to begin the process of deeply understanding the patient and the disease. We are interested in everything about you. The best way we have found to elicit this information is to listen carefully. You, like everyone else, have a story to tell. It is that story that makes you different from others. It is the task of the homeopath to match the pattern of that uniqueness to the pattern of one specific homeopathic medicine.

The medicine which is most similar to your symptoms will have a significant, often dramatic, healing effect. If a homeopath chooses a medicine which is not so similar, usually absolutely no change will occur. Occasionally a medicine that is a close but not an exact match will produce a partial or temporary effect. We are searching for that medicine which has a significant and lasting effect, hopefully resulting in at least a 60 to 70% improvement in your complaints.

In the case of depression, for example, psychiatrists choose between ten or fewer medicines. For the same person with depression, a homeopath will choose among as many as two thousand medicines in order to attain the greatest specificity and most profound results.

Many Substances, Many Dilutions

What are the sources of these medicines that are capable of producing such a deep and long-lasting change in a person's health and well-being? Homeopathic medicines are made from every substance in nature imaginable. The plant, mineral and animal kingdoms are the most common sources for our medicines. Some of the medicines, sometimes called *remedies*, which are used most frequently by homeopaths are made from sulfur, oyster shell, club moss, table salt, honeybee, poison ivy and onion. Natural substances only very recently introduced into the homeopathic repertoire include hydrogen, chocolate, rose, lion's milk, granite and lavender.

Even more unusual than the sources of these medicines is how they are prepared. Hahnemann, the founder of homeopathy, discovered that the greater the dilution, the deeper acting and longer lasting the effect of the medicine. The feature of homeopathy that most stretches the mind and is the biggest obstacle to its acceptance by the mainstream scientific community is the extent to which the medicines are diluted. There are two scales: decimal (dilutions of nine parts of the original substance to one part water or alcohol) and centesimal (ninety-nine to one). We are talking about serial dilutions.

In treating depression and other mental and emotional problems we, as experienced practitioners, most often use preparations of 200C (200 serial dilutions of a centesimal preparation) or 1M (1000 dilutions). In a pharmacy or health food store, you are likely to find 6X (six serial dilutions on a decimal scale) or 30C (30 dilutions of a centesimal). The more dilute, the longer the effect of the medicine.

Classified as over-the-counter drugs, homeopathic medicines are regulated by the Food and Drug Administration. Growing rapidly in popularity, sales of homeopathic medicines have risen recently at a rate of around 20 to 25% a year. (Ullman, 1995, p. 34) Homeopathic pharmacies, which produce the medicines, follow strict guidelines established by the *Homeopathic Pharmacopoeia of the United States*. Some homeopathic preparations are available in pharmacies, health food stores or supermarkets; others are limited to licensed medical practitioners.

How Does Homeopathy Work?

There are a number of plausible hypotheses explaining the action of homeopathic medicines. Although we know that homeopathy does work we cannot explain exactly why or how. This is really no different from our lack of understanding of the mechanism of many pharmaceutical drugs which are nonetheless effective. Nor do we fully understand the effect on brain chemistry of serotonin, dopamine, norepinephrine and the many other neurotransmitters, discovered as well as unknown ones.

There is little doubt that homeopathic medicines, like acupuncture, work on an energetic rather than merely physiological level. In the 19th century, Hahnemann proposed that a homeopathic medicine similar in symptoms to the natural disease from which the person was suffering caused a temporary artificial disease powerful enough to replace the original illness. The medicinal disease, though more powerful than the natural disease, was shorter acting and would disappear in time, leaving the patient well. (Hahnemann, aphorism 29).

Some believe that a type of resonance occurs in which the specific homeopathic medicine vibrates at the same frequency as the constellation of symptoms. This allows the two vibrations to cancel each other out, thus eliminating the disease.

The most exciting explanation of the effectiveness of homeopathic microdoses at this point in time involves the formation of liquid crystals which facilitate the memory of water in which it has been diluted. Recent studies have demonstrated that water, which acts as the medium for most homeopathic medicines, is able to store the memory of antigens and create physiological changes in immune system cells at dilution levels where no chemical substance should remain. (Bellavite, p. 68-78) Some researchers, along this line of thinking, hypothesize that the double-distilled water used to prepare the homeopathic medicines retains the memory of the substance, which was diluted. The highly diluted homeopathic medicines are thus able to produce energetic as well as physiological changes in a human being or animal.

The mystery of the micro-dose continues, and it will take a great deal more research to unravel it. Although homeopathic practitioners and those who have experienced its benefits do not need proof that it does work, skeptics and those unfamiliar to homeopathy may need more evidence to make the leap to try homeopathy or recommend it to others. Until research methodologies are further refined and employed, exactly how homeopathy works will remain an enigma.

Research, Research, Research

Credibility of any therapeutic modality, in the eyes of the scientific community, depends on double-blind studies using a placebo control group. Never mind that the therapy has been shown to have considerable success in treating patients over many years or decades. Even though the conventional wisdom changes its mind frequently about the efficacy of this or that therapy and everyone knows that you can lie with statistics, research is the bottom line. Dana Ullman, M.P.H. (no relation) has worked diligently for decades, compiling the scientific research corroborating the effectiveness of homeopathic medicine. We owe the credit for much of the research that we cite in this section to him and encourage anyone interested in delving more deeply into this material to read his E-book, *Homeopathic Family Medicine: Connecting Research to Quality Homeopathic Care.* (Ullman, 2011)

Funding and human resources for studies testing the efficacy of homeopathy have been limited. Nevertheless, there are a number of well-designed studies, particularly over the past few years, including a meta-analysis conducted at the University of Glasgow, which showed homeopathic medicines to be more effective than a placebo in strengthening the immune system (Reilly, et al., p. 1601). A review of over 100 clinical trials in homeopathy conducted between 1966 and 1990 was published in the *British Medical Journal* in 1991. (Kleijnen, p. 302) The results were positive in 76% of the studies for conditions such as digestive problems, flu, hay fever, rheumatoid arthritis, infections, fibromyalgia, recovery from surgery and psychological problems. Although the authors did not understand how homeopathy actually achieved these results, they recommended more research with better designs. The most favorable article on homeopathy in the scientific literature to date is a recent meta-analysis in the highly respected British medical journal *The Lancet,* which reviewed all 89 of the existing studies on homeopathy (Linde, p. 834-43). The authors concluded that the clinical effects of homeopathy were not due merely to placebo, but that further rigorous and systematic research should be conducted.

Unfortunately, even well documented investigations on homeopathy can be rejected by some at face value simply because they do not believe that homeopathy could possibly work. A famous study by the respected French physician and immunologist Jacques Benveniste tested highly diluted doses of an antibody on a type of white blood cells called basophils. This work, replicated at four different universities, was published, and concurrently refuted, in the prestigious journal *Nature* (Ullman, 1995, p. 58-9) The research proved that the immunoglobulin antibody (IgE) continued to react when exposed to an antigen even after being repeatedly diluted in water. This immune reaction continued even when the water no longer contained even a single mole-cule of antibody according to scientific theory. It was evident that Benveniste was trying to verify the reasoning behind homeopathy. In the same issue, the editors stated that they did not believe the results were true. (Maddox, p. 787) This led to a hot debate in which the editors of *Nature* supported the claims that the research was unfounded. Nevertheless the results were verified a number of times afterwards.

An excellent review of the principles of homeopathy and clinical evidence supporting homeopathy appeared in *Annals of Internal Medicine* in 2003. (Jonas, et al., p. 393-99) A remarkably comprehensive review two years later cited 475 laboratory and clinical trials. (Van Wassenhoven, p. 107-24) Even more interesting and compelling to us that double-blind, placebo-controlled research are the outcomes produced by homeopathic clinicians. One international study involved 30 clinicians in 6 clinics in 4 countries who enrolled 500 consecutive patients with upper respiratory tract complaints, lower respiratory tract complaints or ear complaints. (Riley, Fischer, and Singh, 2002.) 82.6% of patients receiving homeopathic care experienced improvement, while only 68% of those receiving a conventional medication experienced a similar degree of improvement. 67.3% of homeopathic patients experienced improvement with homeopathy within 3 days, while only 56.6% of patients given conventional medicines experienced improvement within that time (16.4% of homeopathic patients improved within 24 hours; 5.7% in other group).

For those wanting to further investigate the controlled studies on homeopathy, we also recommend *Homeopathy: A Frontier in Medical Science* by Paolo Bellavite, MD and Andrea Signorini, MD, a leading Italian pathology professor and a homeopathic physician. After extensive study of the scientific and academic literature on homeopathy, the authors concluded, "The implications of research in homeopathy are very far-reaching. From a general point of view, our very understanding of biological and physiological reality could be greatly extended by it. The phenomenon of the effects of micro-doses, prepared according to homeopathic procedures, may also have spin-off applications in botany, veterinary science, and in the study of ecosystems. In medicine, the specific, rationalized use of small doses (or high dilutions) of specific substances for stimulating or restoring the balance of endogenous defense and repair systems of the human body may complement, increase and even, in some cases, replace the present technological approach." (Bellavite, p. 306) To quote Deepak Chopra, author of *Quantum Healing*, "Medicine is reluctant to walk through the quantum door, even though this experiment [of Benveniste] clearly opens it." (Chopra, p. 114)

"One of the most simple yet sophisticated explanations for how homeopathic doses maintain an active biological effect has been developed by two professors at the University of Arizona, Drs. Gary Schwartz and Linda Russek, and further characterized by two MD/homeopaths, Iris Bell, MD, PhD and David Riley, MD. They postulate the 'systematic memory hypotheses' (Schwartz and Russek, 1999; Schwartz, Russek, Bell, Riley, 2000). They assert that the water retains a memory of the medicinal substance, even after repeated dilutions. Further, they postulate that information and energy (IE) is stored in complex dynamical systems and that 'by reducing the material concentration (the physical dosage) of molecular systems in a diluent (such as water) and at the same time increasing the IE concentration (the IE dosage) in the diluent through repeated succussions (vigorous shakings) leading to increased systemic memory, IE resonance effects may be enhanced' (Schwartz, Russek, Bell, Riley, 2000)." (Ullman, 2011, p. 27)

Scientists at several universities and hospitals in France and Belgium have discovered that the vigorous shaking of the water in glass bottles causes extremely small amounts of silica fragments or "chips" to fall into the water. (Demangeat, Gries, Poitevin, 2004) In fact, these researchers found that high amounts (6 parts per million) of released silica infiltrate the water. These "silica chips" may help to store the information in the water, with each medicine that is initially placed in the water creating its own pharmacological effect. (ibid, 29)

Masaru Emoto, a Japanese researcher who developed the capacity to take photographs of frozen water crystals, has published a number of books showing that water exposed to locations, music, words, prayers, images, symbols and concepts is capable of recording a unique pattern of information in the pattern of the frozen crystals. The ability of water to carry information could be inferred to be a similar process where the information of a particular substance is infused into water molecules, which then could persist through the dilutions and shaking required to produce a homeopathic medicine that can impart that vibration to the watery system of the human body. (Emoto, 1999, 2006)

Despite many advances in modern medicine, the predominating wisdom is still flat-earth. We look forward to further studies whose results are received by an open-minded, unprejudiced and sincerely curious scientific and medical community. There is an international group of homeopathic physicians and other practitioners dedicated to furthering research. As more funding becomes available, we anticipate many more studies over the next decade. We as homeopaths definitely want the documentation, beyond our clinical experience, to understand how and why homeopathy works. As research continues to expand and we are better able to meet the challenges of rigorously demanding scientists, we hope that they, too, will be convinced that homeopathy works.

St. John's Wort Is Not Homeopathy

It is easy to confuse one natural therapy with another, particularly if they are all new to you. Homeopathy is, specifically, the use of homeopathic medicines prescribed according to the philosophy of homeopathy that we have already mentioned. There are many other natural approaches, which are used for depression, anxiety and all kinds of other problems. We want to mention them here both to acknowledge that they can be helpful and also to help you differentiate them from the homeopathic approach that we discuss in this book.

The most well known natural therapy for depression is St. John's wort. Its botanical name is *Hypericum perforatum*. Botanical (herbal) extracts of St John's wort are in widespread use in Germany for the treatment of anxiety, mild to moderate depression and sleep problems. In 1993 more than 2.7 million prescriptions were filled for the most popular preparations of the herb. (Brown-Christopher, p. 23 and Okie, p. E3) More than 20 clinical studies have been completed on the effectiveness of St. John's wort for depression.

"Most have shown the herb to have a greater antidepressant effect than placebo or as great an effect as standard prescription drugs." (Brown, p. 151) The incidence of side effects has varied, from none to 25%, in clinical trials, and they include emotional vulnerability, fatigue, weight gain and itching. (Brown, p. 151) There are also some contraindications while using St. John's wort including the use of over-the-counter cold and flu medications, narcotics, amphetamines and certain foods and alcoholic beverages. (Brown, p. 151) The National Institute of Health, impressed with the potential of the herb, have funded a $4.5 million, three-year study of its effectiveness as compared with a placebo and Zoloft. (Okie, p. E3) St. John's wort as it is being used for depression is a single herb used in its crude, botanical form and is neither prepared or prescribed according to homeopathic indications.

More dietary approaches than we could possibly mention as well as nutritional supplements, such as orthomolecular therapy (high doses of vitamins), tryptophan, D-L phenylalanine, inositol, DMAE and melatonin have been used for depression as has light therapy, negative ions, stress redution and exercise. A number of herbs have been used since ancient times to ease anxiety. The most common are valerian, passion flower, skullcap, hops, catnip and, most recently, kava kava.

Different strokes for different folks. As naturopathic physicians, we are well aware of the importance of diet, exercise and lifestyle on health and well-being and do not doubt that some people are able to alleviate their depression using these methods. We do not elaborate on them in this book because our success has been with homeopathy. Although we encourage our patients to eat fresh, whole, preferably organic food, we have found homeopathy to work regardless of a person's diet. Even though there are many beneficial natural therapies, we have not found one which is as effective as homeopathy not just for mental and emotional problems, but for the whole person.

Homeopathy Around the World

Homeopathic medicine is widely practised worldwide. In France, homeopathy is the most popular type of alternative therapy, is accepted by up to 70% of conventional physicians and is available in every one of the 22,000 or so French pharmacies. Most French pharmacists receive training in homeopathic pharmacology and homeopathic medicines are fully reimbursed by the national health care system. Great Britain also harbors a climate highly favorable to homeopathy. Approximately 42% of British physicians refer patients to homeopathic practitioners, many of whom are covered under the British health care system. Nearly 10% of German physicians specialize in homeopathy and an additional 10% prescribe homeopathic medicines occasionally. Germany also is home to 11,000 *Heilpraktikers*, natural health practitioners, 3,000 of whom specialize in homeopathy. (Dana Ullman, p. 36-7) Homeopathy is also popular in Argentina, Brazil and Mexico.

6 Different Medicines for Different People

Homeopathy Emphasizes the Uniqueness of the Individual

If you are depressed or anxious or you are suffering from any other mental or emotional problem, a homeopath will prescribe a single medicine based on all of your symptoms and unique characteristics. During a lengthy interview in which you are encouraged to speak freely and tell your story in your own words, the homeopath will elicit your life pattern and the particular ways in which you are out of balance. Even the interview itself, when someone listens to you intently for an hour and a half, can be a healing experience. But the real changes will come later, after you are given the correct medicine.

As you read the cases in this book you will see common symptoms running through the stories of depressed and anxious people: sadness, grief, joylessness, worry, fear and apathy to name a few. Although the common symptoms set the stage for allowing the homeopath to know your general features, they do not provide the richness of detail necessary for arriving at a successful homeopathic prescription. As you examine the cases, you will also see that each individual requires a particular homeopathic medicine. This is not to say that no two people will need the same medicine. A single homeopathic medicine may be broad enough in scope to match the illnesses of many different people, or narrow enough to only match a few rare cases. For a given patient at a given time, though, only a single medicine is required to bring about a healing response.

Suppose you meet two people on the street who both seemed depressed, one of whom is your friend Tom, and one of whom is a complete stranger. Both might look dejected, with a slumped posture and sad expression, but you could easily tell which of the two was your friend. You recognize your friend's body type, facial features, hairstyle, tone of voice, mannerisms — a thousand points of recognition that make this person Tom and no one else. It does not matter whether your friend is actually happy or sad at the moment, he is still the one you recognize of these two. The other person will remain a stranger until you meet him, learn his name is Joe, and make observations about the points defining his uniqueness. If you assume because of the way he presents himself that Joe is depressed, you will be wrong. He is actually suffering a temporary bout of influenza that has made him feel absolutely terrible, so he looks sad. Tom, on the other hand, has just lost his job and is in a true, deep depression — and is in fact contemplating suicide.

Homeopaths are experts at differentiating one person from another. Observing Tom and Joe and listening to what they have to say and how they express themselves, homeopaths can glean the necessary details to make a successful homeopathic prescription.

You Are More Than a Diagnosis

In conventional medicine, a diagnosis is made based upon a standard set of observable criteria that delineates a given diagnosis from other similar diagnoses and leads the physician to prescribe a corresponding treatment. For a diagnosis of major depression, for example, you must have experienced five or more of the following symptoms during the same two-week period, including at least one of the first two: depressed mood most of the day, nearly every day; markedly diminished interest or pleasure in all or almost all activities; significant weight loss when not dieting, weight gain or increase or decrease in appetite; too much or too little sleep; agitation or slowness of your activities and responses; fatigue or loss of energy; feelings of worthlessness or inappropriate guilt; diminished ability to think or concentrate, or indecisiveness; and recurrent thoughts of death or suicide. (*Diagnostic and Statistical Manual of Mental Disorders (DSM)* 4th edition, American Psychiatric Association, as cited by Cunningham, p. 401)

What is missing in that method of diagnosis is individualization. "If the patient fulfills the criteria, treatment with antidepressant medication should be considered even if the physician thinks the patient 'has a good reason to be depressed'." (Cunningham, p. 401) If you meet the criteria, you will likely be given a trial of one of several antidepressant medications, such as Prozac, Zoloft, Paxil, Wellbutrin, Effexor, Serzone or Remeron, based on the relative effectiveness of the medication for your observed symptoms and the risks of side effects for you in light of your health history.

For treatment of depression and anxiety, the characteristics in the *DSM* are only a beginning for differentiating which homeopathic medicine will most benefit the patient. Diagnostic criteria in and of themselves are not as important to the homeopath as the individualizing characteristics of the patient. In conventional medicine, patients may be loosely classified as anxious or depressed, phobic, bipolar, schizophrenic, neurotic or obsessive-compulsive. For convenience of communication, homeopaths will use the same terms in describing a patient, but the diagnosis alone does not lead to the homeopathic prescription or treatment protocol. It is the unique, specific characteristics of the patient that are critical to determining the correct medicine. This is even more important for patients who have either been misdiagnosed and therefore mistreated, or whose diagnosis is in question. However, even if they have responded favorably to psychiatric medicines, most people prefer being recognized as unique individuals rather than diagnostic labels.

Little Things Mean So Much

A homeopath wants to know all the details — everything about your health and history that contributes to your present state of ill health and mental and emotional distress. In homeopathy it is often the little facts about you and the way that you feel that make the difference in prescribing one medicine over another.

We want to know how you came to feel the way you do. What life incidents have occurred to produce a recurrent emotional pattern? How, specifically, have you responded to events in the past, emotionally, mentally and physically? What particular thoughts and feelings arise during one of your depressive episodes? How are they the same or different from your usual state? Is there any history of psychological trauma or abuse? What were you like as a child? Does your way of responding resemble your parents' responses in any way? What have been your successes and failures, and how have you responded to them?

The smallest details and the oddest symptoms are often helpful in determining the most appropriate medicine. For example, a person complains of headaches that are their worst at 10 A.M. and most severe from being out in the sunshine. A conventional physician would think, *"So what?"* But to a homeopath it may be the key to finding the correct medicine. When you add to the mix the fact that the person has cold sores on his lips and is depressed over a disappointment in love but feels better after hearing sad music, the homeopathic medicine for the patient becomes crystal clear: *Natrum muriaticum* (sodium chloride). However, if the person has headaches from being in the sun but feels suicidal after hearing music, hates certain kinds of people, is sickened from drinking milk and has very weak ankles, the medicine she needs is *Natrum carbonicum* (sodium carbonate).

Again, it is the small details that can mean so much in figuring out which homeopathic medicine will benefit a person the most.

7 Why Choose Homeopathy to Treat Depression?

Deep, Long-lasting Change Without Drugs

As you will see from the actual cases of real patients in this book, homeopathy produces startlingly positive results in people with psychiatric problems — and many other health problems as well. The right homeopathic medicine stimulates a process of healing that can literally transform a person's life. People who have been depressed for a long time — perhaps even their entire lives — can find renewed hope and develop brighter spirits, more energy and improved physical health. Anxious people find themselves calmer and less worried, their panic relieved. Schizophrenic patients find new order and coherence in their thinking process as delusions and voices recede. The homeopathic process heals the subconscious as well as the conscious mind. Traumatic memories may resurface spontaneously in thoughts, feelings and dreams that lead to resolution and release of psychological pain. Old hurts, griefs, anxieties, injustices, jealousies and obsessions can be put in their proper perspective and released.

The cases presented in this book are of people who have done very well after homeopathic treatment for a wide variety of mental and emotional complaints including grief, depression, low self-esteem, anxiety, phobias and panic attacks, bipolar disorder, schizo-phrenia, dissociative identity disorder and obsessive-compulsive disorder. Although individual case studies do not necessarily prove the effectiveness of treatment, you may find them nonetheless compelling and convincing. Many of our patients certainly feel that they have been helped considerably by their homeopathic treatment.

A Highly Effective Type of Medicine

How well does homeopathy work for depression? Homeopathy is an effective treatment for depression for most people. As we have become more experienced in the practice of homeopathy, we have found that the limits on success are more practical than theoretical. Homeopathic effectiveness is most limited by the skill, knowledge and experience of the homeopath and the cooperation of the patient. The theory works, but it must be applied well and for a long enough time to produce results.

We are able to help a significant number of those who see us, and the results are very gratifying. Often we are able to find the correct medicine after the first interview, but it sometimes takes a number of prescriptions to find the one that works best. In most cases, if both the homeopath and the patient can persevere for six months to a year, a homeopathic medicine will be found that is highly effective. Unfortunately, homeopathy cannot help everyone. There are too many variables involved to promise universal cure, especially with complex psychological disorders. No form of medicine can guarantee that. In addition to the homeopath's skill and experience, you as a patient also play a big role in the homeopathic process by reporting your symptoms accurately and completely, and by following certain guidelines for treatment. (Ullman and Reichenberg-Ullman, p. 57–63)

Safe and Natural

Homeopathic medicine is one of the safest forms of medicine available. It is natural, nontoxic and not addictive. It does not cause side effects in the same way as conventional pharmaceutical drugs, which are chemical substances with direct physiological effects. Homeopathic medicines are energy medicines, which have indirect physiological effects through stimulation of the immune system and other restorative and protective body mechanisms. They are highly diluted chemically, yet quite potent therapeutically. As previously explained, homeopathic medicines are made by serial dilution, and even though the source substance may cause symptoms, the extremely dilute medicine will not usually cause any problem unless it is given far too frequently to a very sensitive person.

The most common reaction to a homeopathic medicine, which occurs in up to 50% of patients, is called an aggravation. This is a temporary worsening of already existing symptoms and usually lasts several days. A return of symptoms the patient had previously can also occur, most commonly lasting four to five days. Aggravations and a return of old symptoms usually are an indication that the correct medicine has been given and will be followed by an amelioration of symptoms.

A Real Deal

Compared to conventional treatment, homeopathic treatment is inexpensive. In the United States, homeopathic treatment is administered on an outpatient basis. At present there are no homeopathic psychiatric hospitals in the United States. A few conventional psychiatrists have switched to homeopathic medicine, but most are not permitted to practise homeopathy in a hospital setting. Although a good homeopath may charge as much as some psychiatrists do, patient visits are usually less frequent and the medicine is very inexpensive. A single dose of homeopathic medicine costs between five and fifteen dollars and may last for weeks or months. In contrast, the average cost of Prozac is eighty-seven dollars per month. Some health insurance covers homeopathic treatment, depending on the license of the practitioner.

8 How Is Homeopathy Different from Conventional Medicine?

A New Paradigm That Makes Sense

Homeopathic treatment is quite different from conventional psychiatric care, using a completely different theory and system of medicine than psychiatry uses. Homeopathy views illness as an imbalance in the basic life energy, or *vital force*, of the person. (Ullman and Reichenberg-Ullman, p. 11) The symptoms of psychiatric illness are generated in an attempt by the person's vital force to restore balance in response to the various factors that cause disease. When the vital force is unable to restore balance and symptoms persist, homeopathy can be of help.

Conventional medicine views mental illness as a chemical imbalance in the brain caused by excesses or deficiencies of neurotransmitters such as serotonin, dopamine, acetylcholine and norepinephrine. Homeopathy recognizes the importance of neurotransmitters but maintains that any particular chemical imbalance is merely an indicator of a deeper imbalance at the level of the vital force. Vitalistic thinking is nothing new; it dates back to Hippocrates in 400 B.C. and to the ancient Asian medical texts. It hypothesizes that there is some type of all-pervasive energy or consciousness responsible for health and healing and that there is more to a person than meets the eye or the microscope. Modern medicine, on the other hand, is based on mechanism and considers the human body-mind as merely a machine. This philosophy views each body as a carefully tuned biological mechanism that is relatively consistent from person to person and that can be thoroughly understood through examination, laboratory testing and dissection.

While homeopaths are interested in understanding a patient's symptoms as an indication of imbalance in the vital force to determine what homeopathic medicine most closely matches it, psychiatrists are interested in understanding how the brain malfunctions in mental illness, and how to rebalance brain chemicals through pharmaceutical intervention. Homeopathy evaluates alterations in mental and emotional states first, then the physical body, acknowledging that the body and mind are not separate. Psychiatry looks first to the function of the brain and body as they alter the mental and emotional state. Both homeopathy and psychiatry seek to produce positive changes in consciousness, attitude, mood, thoughts, emotions and behavior, and to eliminate mental and emotional pathology.

Permanent Change Versus Temporary Palliation

Homeopathic care attempts to provide a permanent change in the person so that mental illness is eventually cured. Although psychiatry would *like* to cure, it generally settles for ongoing drug therapy to maintain a mental state relatively free of symptoms of disorders. Homeopathy usually gives a single microdose of one natural substance, which can last for months or years, needing only occasional repetition if symptoms return. Homeopathy has few side effects, although the presenting symptoms do at times get somewhat worse in the first few weeks of treatment before improvement begins. Conventional psychiatry uses daily doses of chemical drugs, which can have significant, sometimes serious, and even permanent side effects.

Our experience has shown that homeopathic treatment yields more permanent results than psychiatric medications. When taking conventional medications for depression or bipolar disorder or schizophrenia, once you discontinue your medicine(s) — even after years of treatment — symptoms often return immediately, perhaps to a greater degree than before. This indicates that the illness has not been cured, only temporarily managed or suppressed. Once you are treated successfully with homeopathy for a period of months or years, you are less likely to ever relapse fully and should maintain the considerable improvement gained over time. If your symptoms do return, the homeopathic medicine is repeated and the positive effect should again last for a number of months or longer.

57

Discovering the Underlying Cause of Disease

High-technology medicine has made tremendous advances in both diagnosis and treatment. Newer and better drugs are being developed to meet the challenges of human disease, some of which have been very useful and successful, although others have been shortsighted or disastrous failures. Imaging techniques and surgery — such as CAT scans, MRIs, micro-surgery, fiber-optic surgery and open-heart surgery — have become amazingly sophisticated. On the psychiatric front, new generations of antidepressants, tranquilizers and antipsychotic medications are continually being developed. PET scans can tell what areas of the brain are performing various functions and how those change under the influence of pharmaceutical medications.

With all this progress, however, conventional medicine still has no overall theory about why people become sick and how to cure them. Medical techniques come and go, drugs come and go, all supported by research that is eventually superseded or found to have been false. In contrast, homeopathy has a medical theory and practice that empirically work very well and have stood the test of time but whose mechanism of action is still unknown.

Conventional medicine is at its best in surgery, trauma care, life support and management of infectious disease. Homeopathy performs very well with chronic, degenerative disease, acute illness, mental and emotional illness and disease prevention. Each system has its strengths, and in many cases, the two can work together very well.

9 What You Need to Know About Homeopathic Treatment

What to Expect As a Homeopathic Patient

Whether homeopathy is totally new to you or as familiar as your own name, you will be guided in this chapter through any uncharted waters of this unique therapy so that you can reach your goal of improved mental health. There are just a few simple points that will help you understand how to make the most of your homeopathic treatment and avoid any potential problems that may stand in the way of the excellent results possible.

The Patient Who Treats Himself Has a Fool for a Patient

You can benefit a great deal from homeopathy prescribed by someone who knows how, so we advise you to leave the treatment of chronic disease or mental and emotional problems to an expert homeopath. It is too complicated to treat yourself for these kinds of conditions, and your chance of success is not high. Although books exist that give cookbook solutions for complicated mental states, please do not be fooled. We definitely recommend learning to use homeopathy for yourself and your family only for first-aid and acute conditions, according to careful guidelines such as those recommended in our *Homeopathic Self-Care: The Quick and Easy Guide for the Whole Family.* However, for any chronic or recurrent condition — whether physical, mental, or emotional — find the most qualified person or persons to help you.

The Homeopathic Interview

You will have an initial consultation with your homeopath, either in person or, if there is no experienced practitioner in your area, through telephone consultation. You may be surprised by how much time a homeopath will allow to take your case history, especially during your initial interview. For adults, a first visit usually lasts an hour or more, and for children, at least an hour. During this time, the homeopath will take your case history and perform any necessary physical examinations (which can be performed locally by another doctor in the case of telephone consultation). The case history is very extensive and designed to discover the unique pattern of symptoms that determines which homeopathic medicine will work best for you. It will cover your complete mental and emotional state, as well as any physical health problems you may have. Your life situation, likes and dislikes, food preferences, temperature and weather tolerance, even the position in which you sleep will be explored. You may wonder why the homeopath needs to know this information, but it is all crucial to determining the specific homeopathic medicine for you. You will probably share thoughts with your homeopath that you have not told anyone. You can be sure that they will be held in the utmost confidentiality.

The interview is set up to allow you to tell your story with a minimum of interference, distraction and unnecessary questioning. Just say whatever comes to mind about yourself, your life, your nature as a person, your emotional state and any problems you have been having mentally and physically. You may think you are just rambling, but your homeopath will be busy putting the pieces together into a coherent pattern. She is observing, listening and taking pages of notes while you speak. You will be given the space to speak as much as you like about what has been going on with you.

Your mental and emotional states are particularly important parts of any case history, particularly if your main problem is a psychological one, such as depression, mood swings or anxiety. It may seem like psychotherapy, as the homeopath hones in on your characteristic thoughts and feelings, but the intent is different. What he is doing is matching your mental symptoms with those that are characteristic of certain homeopathic medicines.

The responses you have had to traumatic or abusive experiences, significant life changes, losses and griefs, joys and sorrows, relationship problems, shame, embarrassment, successes and failures can all point to certain homeopathic medicines. Anything that has contributed to a person's mental state may be important. Fears and phobias, anxiety, anger, obsessions and compulsions, peculiar habits, delusions, hallucinations and unusual ways of thinking are all components of one's mental state, which can help point to a particular homeopathic medicine. Any mental or emotional symptom that limits you is important. Each symptom is a thread woven into a tapestry that reveals your nature and the medicine that will help you.

Physical symptoms are also intertwined in the fabric and can sometimes be the deciding factor in choosing between two medicines. Even if you are being treated primarily for depression and anxiety, be sure to tell your practitioner about your physical pains, problems and limitations because homeopathy treats the whole person. Mention anything about yourself that might be considered quirky, peculiar, strange or unusual. These characteristics provide clues for unlocking the door to your healing.

A Prescription for Homeopathic Success

The most important steps that you can take to ensure treatment success are to honestly share what is going on with you and to follow your homeopath's instructions. Clear communication is an important component of any healing relationship; this is especially true with homeopathy. Your practitioner will prescribe a particular medicine to be taken once or at given intervals and will let you know when you need to return for further evaluation.

There are a few substances most homeopaths will ask you to avoid during treatment. These may include coffee and coffee-flavored products (but not all caffeinated substances). You will also be asked to avoid contact with strong aromatic substances, such as camphor and eucalyptus. Your homeopath will offer very specific recommendations. If you are asked to avoid certain things, it is because these factors have been known to interfere with or act as an antidote to homeopathic medicines; they are not being excluded arbitrarily.

The Course of Treatment

After the initial interview, and perhaps after some additional review of your case, your homeopath will select a single medicine and give it to you to take in either a single dose or, occasionally, in multiple doses, depending on what other medications you may be taking or how often it is appropriate. Homeopathic medicines are usually dissolved in the mouth or under the tongue. In many cases only a single high-potency dose is needed to start the healing process. It may need repetition only once in several months or longer.

Your progress will be reviewed in five to eight weeks to see how the medicine has affected you and what has changed since you began the medicine. Usually about thirty minutes are sufficient for a follow-up visit. If you are doing well, you will be asked to continue taking the medicine or to wait for further results if you have been given a single dose. If you have not improved, your homeopath will attempt to determine why the medicine did not work as expected. Sometimes the medicine has no effect whatsoever and another must be selected. Other times the medicine is correct but something has interfered with the healing process.

After the correct medicine has been found for you, your depression, anxiety, grief, mood swings or other symptoms should begin to lessen within three to six weeks. If your homeopath uses single doses, as we do, you will not need an additional dose of the homeopathic medicine as long as progress continues. If you are on conventional medication when you start treatment, we find that it is usually best to continue this along with the homeopathy, sometimes administered in more-frequent low-potency doses — at least until you notice a substantial improvement. At that point, you can consult with the prescribing physician or psychiatrist regarding a safe schedule to reduce or discontinue your chemical medication.

If you are taking drugs for bipolar disorder or schizophrenia, however, you may need to continue taking them indefinitely.

Follow-up appointments with your homeopath to review your progress will usually be about every six to twelve weeks, depending on your progress. As your health improves, the appointments become less frequent. Eventually you may need to be seen only once or twice a year, or on an as-needed basis. If you experience a return of your previous symptoms, your homeopath will want you to come back earlier to make an adjustment in the medicine.

If your symptom picture changes considerably, you may need a different medicine. If you contract an acute illness, such as a sore throat, cough, bladder infection or earache, be sure to consult your homeopath, either prior to consulting your medical doctor or as soon as possible afterward. Acute homeopathic treatment is often very effective and may preclude the need for conventional medications, which in some cases may interfere with your homeopathic treatment.

The Long Haul

When you begin homeopathic treatment, particularly for mental or emotional illness, plan to be committed to the process for at least one to two years. You may see definite improvement within a few weeks of treatment, but it takes time for your body and mind to stabilize in the new pattern. You may need several doses of medicine over the first year or so of treatment to achieve stable progress. It may also take a number of different medicines and up to six months or more to find the best one for you. Do not give up easily on homeopathic treatment or you will miss out in the long run. We estimate that at least 70% of those patients who stay in treatment for a year or more will improve significantly. Most experienced homeopaths will be able to find an effective medicine for you over time, and quite often within the first two to four months of treatment. You may need a rare or unusual medicine that cannot be determined until the more common medicines have been used first, or once your homeopath knows you better or additional information may suggest a change in medicine.

If you are frustrated by a lack of progress and you are not getting sufficient relief from your symptoms, talk this over with your practitioner. Perhaps a consultation with or referral to a more experienced homeopath is in order.

Different Kinds of Homeopaths

When we say to try a different homeopath, we are still speaking about classical homeopaths, who take a full case history, give one homeopathic medicine at a time, and wait for weeks or months to assess the result. Other kinds of practitioners may use the term *homeopath*, or *homeopathic physician*, and mean something totally different. If your practitioner focuses primarily on nutrition, vitamins and cleansing programs, she is probably not specializing in classical homeopathy. If you are diagnosed by a machine or by muscle testing rather than by interview and examination, you are not being treated by a classical homeopath. This is not to say that these other practitioners may not also be using homeopathic medicines or may not be effective in treating your problem. They are simply doing something other than what we are describing in this book.

It is best if your homeopath has taken more than one thousand hours of training, with clinical experience included. Many homeopaths already have a medical license of some kind, acquiring most or all of their homeopathic education through postgraduate courses and seminars. There is also a growing number of qualified, unlicensed homeopathic practitioners. Board certification is an excellent criterion for selection of your homeopath. Directories of homeopaths throughout the United States are available (see the appendix for more information). If you have any doubt as to the experience, qualifications or style of practice, inquire prior to scheduling your first appointment.

10 Practical Tips to Deal with Depression, Anxiety and Other Emotional Problems

Tips to Make Your Life Fuller, Happier and Healthier

Be Here Now

The only moment you need to attend to right now is the present one. We waste valuable time and energy worrying about the future, which is merely a figment of our imaginations, or dwelling on the past, which is history. We have absolutely no idea what will occur in the next moment, much less the next year or decade. Live each day to the fullest and enjoy it heartily — as if it were your last. If today was not what you wanted it to be, move on and create a better tomorrow.

Ask Yourself What Is Truly Important to You

Values help you decide whether what you are doing is worth the price you are paying. What would you save from your burning home and what wouldn't you care about? If this were the last year of your life, what would you do with it? What do you want people to say about you when you are no longer here? What are the top ten things in your life? What do you most care about doing? Learning? Experiencing? Eating? Feeling? Loving? Find out and do those things, learn those things, experience, eat, feel and love those things. Do what makes your heart sing. Live a passionate life. Make sure how you spend your time reflects what you want out of your life.

Do Your Best Then Let Go

One of the greatest sources of unhappiness is perfectionism. It's the never-good-enough syndrome. You may as well give up trying to be perfect because you will not succeed. Try instead to just be yourself. You are a unique, special individual with a potential and a purpose. Do the best you can in every moment and trust that others are doing the same. It was not an accident that you were born, even if it may sometimes appear that way. The greatest contribution that you can make is to be yourself and to make the most of your gifts and talents.

Don't Sweat the Small Stuff

As Richard Carlson wisely advises in *Don't Sweat The Small Stuff*, most of our worries are not worth the time of day. Prioritize. Take care of what is really important and do the rest when you can, or forget about it. Drop obsessing over the miniscule details of life. It simply isn't worth it. In the long run, no one will care, even you. Know what you can change and let go of the rest. And don't let anything or anyone rob you of your peace of mind.

Take Responsibility

Whether you are responsible for a big or little piece of the world, take full responsibility for it. Take care of whatever is yours to do. No excuses, no blaming others. No manipulating others to do your job for you. If you make a mistake, accept it, apologize and fix it or make it better if you can. What you don't take responsibility for in your life will fall on the shoulders of someone else and you will lose your independence and freedom in the bargain.

Wherever You Go, There You Are

There's only one person who will be your constant companion. You guessed it— it's yours truly. Self-respect is an essential component of happiness. Take time to appreciate all of the positive things about yourself. Give yourself credit for all of the good decisions, the kind thoughts and acts, and the accomplishments that you've achieved, however small. Give yourself a break just as you would give slack to someone else. We all have our rough edges to be ground by the tumbler of life. Take time to appreciate what is good and beautiful inside of you.

And make a commitment to work on whatever you would like to change.

Bad Things Happen to Good People

Life happens. People are born, mature, grow old and die. They are sick and they are well, devastated and elated. It's how we handle the events in our lives that determine our state of mind. We recently heard an Indian sage remark, "acceptance is cure". This means that once we acknowledge the reality of our situation, we are free to act in whatever way we choose to deal with it.

Shortly after we began writing the first edition of this book, in 1998, Judyth, just before her fiftieth birthday, was diagnosed with a slow-growing, non-invasive breast cancer. Within two weeks of her diagnosis, Bob's cousin, John, forty-six years old, was found to have an extremely aggressive brain tumor. In both cases, the illness provided valuable lessons and gathered tremendous love and support of friends and family. Judyth chose surgery, found an excellent and supportive team of practitioners, and was able to find many reasons to be grateful for the experience, despite the shock, the pain and the scars. The cancer served as a wakeup call to reassess what was most important to her.

John's cancer ended very differently. He was quickly bedridden and slipped away within three months. The entire family was drawn together by John's selflessness and sweet surrender. They learned of the many ways that John had helped more people than they had ever known. How he did not ever refuse anyone who turned to him for anything. His bittersweet death, though tragically early, was a reminder to say that we are here to love, pure and simple.

At the same time, we learned that an old friend, Patty, has been diagnosed with a stage four malignant melanoma. The mother of three girls under fourteen, she could feel bitter and resentful, but she doesn't. Instead she is filled with gratitude for all those who are there to help and with prayer that she may be healed. As she receives her radiation treatments, she chooses to look up at the ceiling and imagines all of the thoughts and prayers sent upwards each day by patients just like her. There is nothing she wants more than to be healthy and to see her children blossom into adulthood. Yet she humbly and gracefully accepts each moment as it comes.

Life is full of surprises, some apparently wonderful, others terrible. However, even those circumstances that seem the most grim can later prove to bring wonderful blessings.

Laugh and Smile

In every tragedy lies the seed of an equivalent comedy. Look for the humor and irony in the drama of your life. Laugh about your trials and misfortunes. It makes the sorrows easier to take. Step outside yourself and see what is funny, ridiculous or absurd about your situation. Watch comedy routines and slapstick videos. Hang out with little children, puppies and kittens. They're good for lightening the heart. It's very hard to feel depressed while you're telling a good joke.

Be Honest with Yourself and Others

The old proverb, "Oh what a tangled web we weave when first we practise to deceive" is very true. Being honest builds trust, friendship, relationship and is good business as well. Lying does the opposite. There is no such thing as a white lie. There is some good in sparing someone's feelings through tact and diplomacy, but only if your withholding or softening the truth is really for his or her benefit. Lying, denying and rationalizing will bring unhappiness and mistrust to you and anyone around you. Face your problems, be real about them and find solutions. Be true to yourself.

Be Kind and Generous

The more you devote yourself to helping others, in whatever way you can, the happier you will be and the more you will forget about your own problems. Service to others is service to God and ultimately to yourself. It feels good, it does good, and it makes others feel good, too. Kindness and compassion for others will help you to feel good about yourself and what you are doing in life. Volunteer for what needs doing. Treat others as they would like to be treated, or at least as well as you want to be treated. If you don't know what someone else wants or needs, just ask. We are all in this life together, so we might as well help each other get through it more easily.

Ask for Help When You Need It

Everyone needs a hand now and then, especially when they are feeling blue or upset. Don't be afraid to ask for help if you really need it. It makes people feel good if they can help you over the rough spots, as long as that is not all the time. Love and support are the most valuable gifts, especially during the hard times of life. Don't be an island unto yourself. If you do not have the good fortune of being able to call on friends or family, contact a religious or support group. You'll find that others are very willing to lend you a hand and you'll make good friends in the process. At some other time, when you are feeling up and have some energy, return the favor by helping someone else who is less fortunate or able than you are.

Keep Good Company

Surround yourself with positive, supportive people who believe in you and want you to be happy and to fulfill your dreams. We all need cheerleaders to encourage us through the joys and trials of life. On the other hand, some people can just drag you down or tempt you into destructive or addictive behaviors so they can feel better than you. If you feel yourself caught in a negative spiral down and surrounded by people who are sinking just like yourself, it is time to find some new companions. Keeping good company helps you to be inspired and to fulfill your highest potential.

Cultivate an Attitude of Gratitude

Even at the glummest and most distressing of times, remember all the things for which you can be grateful. Give thanks for the little things that brighten your day and give meaning to your life. Give thanks for the big things that support and nourish your well-being — a roof over your head, food to sustain you, the air you breathe, the water you drink. Give thanks to the people in your life who are there for you. Give thanks to your parents, wife, children, relatives and friends just for being. Give thanks to your supporters, helpers and caregivers. Thank God for giving you life and make the most of it.

Heal The Relationships That You Can and Release the Others, Forgive and Forget

Even the kindest, most conscious person makes mistakes and acts in ways that are hurtful to others, intentionally or not. These hurts turn into grievances between individuals and wars between nations. Take stock of any times that you have been hurt or have hurt others, any time in your lives, then forgive yourself and ask forgiveness of those other individuals. The amount of suffering which can be released through forgiveness is tremendous.

Make amends with those you have hurt and forgive those who have hurt you. Sometimes, it is possible and sometimes it is not, but it is often necessary to make the attempt to heal past relationship problems if you want to feel good in the present. Apologizing and forgiving can be the most powerful vehicles to heal or transform a relationship or even a life. A great deal of the emotional baggage we carry has to do with unhealed relationships. The negativity you hold on to can backfire and make you sick. We have seen many patients whose illnesses were fueled by bitterness and resentment. The hardest thing may be letting it go, but it is for the best. Try to feel compassion for those who have hurt you, because they were obviously too ignorant or in pain to do any better. Remember also, when you have been the hurtful one, to step outside yourself and feel compassion for your own ignorance and pain, too. Be sure to thank yourself and the other person for demonstrating the vulnerability and courage to let go and move forward.

Eat Well

The better you eat, the better you feel. Nutritious, live, natural food, supported by high quality nutritional supplements, will give your body what it needs to make energy, give you strength and vitality and keep you healthy and happy. Eat a colorful diet of whole, fresh, attractive, nourishing food, organic food — fresh fruits and vegetables; whole grains; olive oil, wild salmon and other cold-water fish sources of Omega-3; nuts and seeds, including walnuts, almonds and flax seed, and drink lots of water. Taste fresh chicken eggs with deep yellow yolks and you won't want the store-bought variety again. Be vegetarian or eat farm-raised, and white and red meat. If you enjoy dairy products, don't overdo them. Eat sugar only as a special treat and drink alcohol in limited quantities, except for red wine. A steady diet of junk and fast food is nearly devoid of any vitamins and minerals or fiber.

Burn Those Calories

You'd be surprised how your mood will lift once you engage in regular, vigorous exercise. Take a deep breath, fill your lungs deeply with fresh air, and feel your red blood cells celebrate. Pick an activity that you enjoy, or that you used to enjoy, and make it a daily, or nearly, routine. Get a trainer to help you set up your workouts. Feel those muscles getting healthier by the day. Walk in a local park, in the woods or even around the block, do jumping jacks, jog, work out, play tennis, shoot a few hoops, swim, swing a golf club, dance. Do anything to get up, out and moving around. Your body and mind will be very happy and those endorphins will lift your spirits.

Stretch Your Body

Stretching your body every day, either through yoga or any other method that works for you, will keep you far more healthy and comfortable for many years. We have observed that many folks, as they age, begin to move around with great discomfort and pain. Joint and muscle pain are no fun and can put a real damper on your mobility, enjoyment and quality of life. There are classes for every age and experience level. Whether you do your stretches with others or on your own, don't let a day pass without a good, long stretch.

Slow Down

Some of our anxieties and worry come from doing too much and not taking enough time to process it. Things just seem to move too fast, there is too much to do and to think about. We are on information overload. It is overwhelming at times! Take some time to slow down. If you are in the city, go to the country for a week or a weekend. Turn off your cell phone, your fax machine, your computer, e-mail and voice mail. Walk instead of drive to the store. Ride a bicycle. Take a break from TV, radio and newspapers. Simplify your life and watch your anxiety diminish.

Breathe In, Breathe Out

The easiest, quickest way to change you mood and attitude is through your breath. What's most important is to relax, breathe slowly and deeply, and let your worries and thoughts dissolve. One technique that can be done anywhere and anytime is alternate nostril breathing. Find a comfortable place where you won't be disturbed. Sit in a comfortable position with your back straight. Hold your right elbow at a forty-five degree angle, press your right nostril closed with your right thumb and gently breathe in through the left nostril to the count of four. Then use your right ring finger to close your left nostril, release the thumb, and, with the elbow still raised, exhale through your right nostril for four counts. Continue for up to five minutes. You can do this when you are feeling upset, uptight, tired or anxious or at bedtime, if you have trouble falling asleep. It will bring a sense of peace and balance. With more experience, you can slow the breath and increase the duration of the exercise. It will help you to find the calm center inside of you and to release fears, worries and unhappiness.

Quieting the Mind

Our busy lives rarely allow us to find the quiet calmness that resides within each of us. It is amazing how quickly we can move from hustle and bustle to deep peace if we just take the time to do so. Whether you relax through relaxation, meditation, contemplation, prayer or walking through nature, allow yourself time to do so every day. Let go of preoccupations, obsessions, catastrophising and self-concern, for at least a few moments, and just be. Once your mind is still, your troubles will seem much less important.

Peace Is the Greatest Gift of All

Nearly everyone wants peace, peace with others and peace within oneself. Peace can be elusive, but it is really with us all the time. We just cover it over with other feelings. If you want to be peaceful, let go of what you are holding onto and be at peace with whatever is happening in the present moment. Be still, close your eyes, take a deep breath. Then another. Be at peace with others. Have no expectations. Your experience may be pleasurable or painful, but you can be sure it will not last forever. Peace is found right now, in the present. Not later, not after you have done something else, or after things get better. Right now. Take a moment, now, clear your mind, forget about the past or the future, your hurts, sorrows and troubles, your joys, aspirations and achievements. Let go. Just breathe. Just be. That is where you will find the peace you seek, this moment and every moment, without effort, within you all the time.

Make Friends with Nature

Urban dwellers often lose touch with the joys of being in nature. Go outside, look at the flowers and trees, walk through a park, listen to the birds sing. Catch the sunrise or the sunset. Gaze at the stars at night. Listen to the waves crash against a rocky shore. Take a hike, climb a mountain, take a dip in an alpine lake, stand at the foot of a glorious waterfall. Communicate with and be kind to animals and plants. Fill your lungs with fresh air. Nature gives us a perspective on how we fit into the grand scheme of things and teaches us what is really important.

Grow a Garden

How refreshing and revitalizing to get your hands in some good, old-fashioned dirt. Enrich your soul as you enrich the soil. Plant organic seeds and marvel at the wondrous vegetables and glorious flowers that soon break through the ground. Admire the rainbow and cornucopia of Mother Nature as reflected in a gorgeous, bright-red carrot or a beautiful purple kale or the endless variations of luscious salad greens. Pick your mouth-watering berries and veggies straight off the vines. Keep a vase of beautiful, freshly cut daisies or dahlias or perfume-scented roses by your bed. It is hard to feel depressed when you admire and ingest plants that are so bursting with life!

Get a Pet

There is nothing more unconditionally loving than a loyal, furry companion. You have probably heard about the various studies about the elderly who are ill, either living at home or in a nursing home, who have domestic pets. They remain healthier and live longer, happier lives. A heartwarming, purring kitty lying happily on your pillow at night or the soulful eyes and happy licks of a canine buddy can do wonders to brighten your day. *Chicken Soup for the Pet Lover's Soul* recounts story after story of people who were healed, inspired and transformed by members of the animal kingdom.

A friend of ours, Amelia Sahentara, wrote a lovely poem which we would like to share: (Sahentara, p. 41)

A Healing Place

This Place

There is a place
where each of us lives without unresolved conflict,
in total honesty and complete sincerity.
It is safe to love without holding back
because there are no divisive judgments
or unacknowledged feelings.
All that needs saying is said.
All that needs hearing is heard.
All that needs mending is mended.
The joy of this place may be felt in the
wee hours of the night when we listen to
our hearts beat in the stillness.
Or it may be seen in the eyes of those
healed of a life-threatening illness.
And it can always be sensed beneath
the drama of our lives and in our dreams,
for there lies the power and mystery of life itself.
This place is like the stars
that shine brightly all through the day
even though our eyes cannot see them.
This place.

11 The Interface Between Homeopathy and a Conventional Approach to Mental Health

For Psychiatrists, Psychologists, Psychotherapists and Other Mental Health Professionals

The many cases in this book are all true stories. Whether or not you believe in homeopathy or in any form of natural medicine, we believe you will agree that many of our patients have experienced a dramatic improvement in their lives. Some of you will insist that all of these changes are the result of placebo — of simply wanting to improve. We don't deny that there may be some placebo effect occurring, but there is much more. A homeopath carefully documents at each visit any change in the patient's mind, body or emotions. If we have not selected the correct medicine, little to no change will occur despite any wishes of the patients and ourselves. We see this regularly in our practice and have mentioned cases in our book where the first or second medicine resulted in no remarkable change. In addition, there is a growing body of research to document that homeopathic medicine does not act merely as a placebo.

We ask you to consider the possibility that there is an effective approach to mental and emotional problems other than conventional medicine and psychotherapy. If this book or other experiences have made you aware of another possibility, why not encourage, or at least observe, a few of your patients who are using homeopathy in addition to your own care. The worst that a patient can lose with homeopathy is time and money. We have not seen any patients mentally or emotionally harmed by homeopathy, as long as the practitioner is experienced, reputable and does not take on patients beyond his or her expertise. As you will see from the cases in this book, many people benefit a great deal from homeopathic care.

Homeopathy and Psychotherapy: A Happy Marriage

Many of our patients have already engaged in psychotherapy, sometimes for many years, before they have consulted us. Some are concurrently consulting us and their psychotherapists. Homeopathy often allows patients to progress more quickly, gain deeper insights and make better use of their therapy time. We do not hesitate to refer our patients for psychotherapy, medical hypnosis, bodywork or any other therapy that might be worthwhile. Sometimes a homeopathic medicine by itself will be enough to catapult the patient into deep transformation. Often homeopathy works in combination with other therapeutic or lifestyle approaches. We suggest, however, that an individual begin only one new approach at a time so that it is possible to clearly evaluate the effect.

If you are seeing a patient for therapy who is also being treated with homeopathy and it is new to you, we suggest that you read our first book, *The Patient's Guide to Homeopathic Medicine*, in order to familiarize yourself with the process of homeopathic treatment.

Can Homeopathy Be Dangerous to Patients with Serious Mental Illness?

We do *not* recommend that a patient taking conventional medicines discontinue the medications prior to beginning homeopathy. The most common fear of health professionals unfamiliar with natural medicine is that it will prevent a truly sick person from getting the treatment that he or she needs. Our approach is not either-or. When necessary and appropriate, we suggest that patients consult a psychiatrist for medications or hospitalization or contact a crisis line. We are seeking a gentle, lasting cure. We would much more prefer steady healing over months or years to a temporary amelioration followed by a relapse.

How Can One Dose of a Homeopathic Medicine Last for Months or Years?

Once an individual has been given a homeopathic medicine that has had a definite positive effect, the improvement generally continues for a minimum of several months — often longer — before it needs to be repeated. It is not really a matter of a pharmacological half-life or how long the medicine stays in the body. It is, rather, a matter of a homeopathic medicine catalyzing a process of healing and change. That process will continue as long as it has momentum. The action of a particular medicine can stop if the patient is exposed to one of the influences that interferes with homeopathic treatment, such as a severe trauma or stress or an acute illness.

How long a dose of a homeopathic medicine lasts depends on many factors, including the vitality of the individual, the duration and severity of the symptoms, environmental stresses and exposures, and whether or not the patient is taking other medications. Some practitioners use a daily or weekly dose of homeopathic medicine in addition to infrequent stronger doses. The most important factors are to understand the patient and to find a homeopathic medicine that is the best match for that patient. The prescribing style of the individual practitioner is secondary.

Will Homeopathy Interfere with the Medications That You Prescribe?

Homeopathic medicines do not diminish the effect of prescription medications. However, when they are effective, the patient's need for psychiatric medication may be diminished or eliminated. We often find that once we have found the best homeopathic medicine for a patient, it is possible for them to work with the prescribing physician over time to lower the dose of their conventional medication with no adverse effects. Frequently, as the patient continues to feel well with homeopathic treatment, it becomes possible for that medication to be discontinued and for the patient to continue to feel well, often even better than with the medication.

Patients who are depressed or anxious sometimes respond very quickly to homeopathic treatment and can work with their psychiatrists or physicians to taper off their other medications within weeks or months. For bipolar patients, it may take several years before they are stable enough to discontinue their lithium, or they may need to continue taking it, along with their homeopathic medicine, indefinitely. Patients suffering from anxiety, even though they are responding well to homeopathy, may wish to take a period of months before giving up their antianxiety medications. Schizophrenic patients being treated with homeopathy and conventional medicine may or may not be able to discontinue the antipsychotics. Our most successful treatment with schizophrenia is often with those patients who have had only one psychotic break and are not caught in the revolving door of psychotropic medications and hospitalization.

Are There Patients Who Cannot Be Helped with Homeopathy?

As with any treatment modality, homeopathy is not for everyone. A patient needs to be committed to following the course of homeopathic treatment. This means at least one year of treatment, often more. Even though homeopathy can promote a rapid and positive response, those looking for a quick fix should look elsewhere.

Patients who have an extensive history of serious mental illness, such as schizophrenia — and are non-compliant about taking medications — are usually not good candidates for homeopathic treatment. An individual must be willing to take responsibility for themself and their actions, to keep scheduled appointments and to communicate openly with the homeopath. Those who are chemically dependent, untruthful in conveying their history, unwilling to avoid exposures that can interfere with homeopathic treatment or unable to provide the information that a homeopath needs have a more guarded prognosis.

When Is It Time to Give Up on Homeopathy and Try Another Approach?

Just as one psychiatrist is not for everyone, the same is true for homeopaths. Areas of expertise, style, personalities and fees are all factors that may make one homeopath a better match than another for a particular patient. Generally it is best to find an experienced homeopathic practitioner and continue with treatment for a year before giving up. Since a homeopath often waits six to eight weeks to evaluate the effect of one medicine before changing it, if necessary, after a year a patient may have taken at most six to eight different medicines. After that period of time, if there has been no significant and lasting response, it may be time to find another homeopath or a different form of therapy. It is important to point out, however, that even experienced practitioners — especially with challenging patients — can take even two or three years to find the medicine that will have the deepest and most lasting effect.

PART III

Successful Homeopathic Treatment of Depression: Our Patients' Stories

12 Can I Live Without Him?

Moving Through and Beyond Grief and Loss

We are born, we live, we love, we die. These are unavoidable human experiences. Along with human relationships come what some call bonding or connection, what others call attachment. Whether a relationship lasts only hours or it endures for decades, intense and lasting interactions and enmeshment occur. Inevitably, due to capriciousness, changing circumstances, illness, divorce, death or destiny, relationships end or at least change in form. This often results in pain on the part of one or both members of the relationship. In some cases, the individual is able to grieve for a period of months and then move forward with their life. Not that the memories or caring are forgotten, but life goes on. Others remain frozen and paralyzed by grief and devastation, incapacitated and unable to continue with the flow of their lives as they knew them before.

Some relationships are terminated abruptly, such as when a loved one is killed prematurely in an automobile accident or a plane crash. All parties are caught off guard and left with the feeling of shock, unpreparedness and unfinished communication. Even lingering or expected deaths can leave the survivors numb, grief stricken and at loose ends. Divorce brings its own type of pain, disbelief, resentment and struggle. The death of a child can be one of the most heart-wrenching tragedies of life. Tremendous suffering can also occur after a miscarriage, stillbirth or abortion. After such losses, the sadness and heartbreak that remain — sometimes for years or even a lifetime — can often be helped dramatically with homeopathic treatment, as shown in the following cases. People sometimes ask whether homeopathy interferes with the normal grieving process. No, it simply helps to bring the individual back into balance and move on with life. It does not prevent the person from experiencing or processing the pain and loss in an honest and healthy way.

"My Daughter Drowned": A Case of Depression and Obsessive-Compulsive Disorder

Barbara, a thirty-five-year-old Los Angeles interior decorator in business with her sister, had been taking Zoloft for two years. Four years before we met her, Barbara's two-year-old daughter, Chelsea, fell into their swimming pool and drowned while she and her husband were at home. Needless to say, she was devastated by the loss of her daughter. Without the help of Zoloft, she felt very afraid that her six-year-old son, Ben, or another child in her care, might be hurt. Before her daughter died, Barbara loved to entertain and was a marvelous cook. After Chelsea's tragic death, Barbara began to worry that her food was unsafe and as a precaution she started throwing out any leftovers. Her concern became so exaggerated that she needed to go shopping for groceries daily. She found it simpler for her family to eat most of their dinners at restaurants.

Life was no longer worth living for Barbara. Despite being a devout Episcopalian, she wished her life would end. The pain of losing Chelsea felt unbearable. Even greater than her sorrow was overwhelming guilt. There was a gate around the pool, but the padlock had been left unlocked. Barbara blamed herself unmercifully for her precious daughter's accident. Prozac had reduced her despair and suicidal feelings, but she discontinued it because it made her anxious.

This was the second time Barbara had felt a tremendous burden of guilt. The first was after an abortion in her late teens. There was no one she could tell — not her parents, not her boyfriend. She felt she had made the decision in opposition to her own beliefs and that she would have to answer for it later. Convinced that her life would not be the same again, the secret of having chosen an abortion tormented her for years. Her terrible self-blame again reared its head following Chelsea's death. Barbara told us that she felt as if she, too, died the moment her daughter fell into the pool.

When asked if there were any other times earlier in her life that she had felt guilt or shame, Barbara recounted that at the age of six an uncle molested her twice and swore her to secrecy. This led to a recurrent series of bladder infections and, since it happened while she was in bed, to insomnia. Even as an adult, Barbara still worried about someone coming into her room at night.

"There's nothing worse than losing a child," Barbara lamented. "Especially a little girl who is so wanted and was the light of our lives. To live with the guilt of being parents and not keeping your child safe ... it's hard to face people." Around the anniversary of Chelsea's death, Barbara felt as if she were "sinking lower and lower." "I give things away to make up for my mistake. I've gotten our family into a lot of debt."

Barbara shared more about her obsessive tendencies. "I was washing my hands excessively because I felt terrified of germs and AIDS. I just couldn't get my hands clean enough. I've been this way since I was six." We remembered that this was when the sexual abuse occurred and asked Barbara how she felt about that experience. "I felt dirty. Like slime. I didn't understand why it happened to me. My report cards mentioned that I had a constant obsession about going to the bathroom, even three times during an hour. I'm still like that." Two years of psychotherapy had been supportive but had not fundamentally shifted Barbara's state of mind for the better.

Barbara's son, Ben, also felt guilty about Chelsea's death. "My husband and I felt so unworthy about living after the accident, yet we knew that we had to provide a stable atmosphere for Ben even though our whole world had blown apart. That first year after it happened I felt like I was in a fog. I wasn't present at all. I was terrified that we would be found negligent and that someone would take Ben away from us.

"During that time I was terrified of AIDS. Any sneeze or cough scared me to death. None of our friends understood what we went through. I felt that I couldn't trust them. But my husband came through for me whenever I needed him. After Chelsea died, he told me I was a wonderful mom and that he wouldn't have wanted anyone else to be the mother of our kids."

Barbara was afraid of being alone and of something happening to her husband. She dreamed of being attacked. Her dreams had become more vivid and strange while she was taking Prozac. Zoloft caused her to have disturbing dreams about unhappy relationships and breakups. Without the Zoloft, Barbara could not fall asleep until 2 A.M.

Acne rosacea and alopecia (loss of hair) were Barbara's physical complaints. She loved starchy food and had a compulsive addiction to caramels. She disliked seafood.

We prescribed for Barbara *Kali bromatum* (potassium bromate). This is an important homeopathic medicine for family-oriented people who often have a rather strict upbringing. Guilt and shame, often about some terrible wrong they believe they have done, torment them. They often feel so bad about their actions that they believe they will receive punishment from God. They often carry a tremendous burden throughout their lives.

Three weeks later Barbara felt so good that, with the consent of her psychiatrist, she stopped taking her Zoloft. "We just went through a very hard anniversary. My depression and suicidal tendencies have been very much in check. I feel really encouraged. The obsessive-compulsive disorder is pretty much under control. I'm doing surprisingly well with the guilt. I'm not feeling burdened by it anymore. I miss Chelsea dreadfully, but I don't feel dragged down. I can finally talk about the accident. I haven't had those feelings of not wanting to be here."

We received a phone call from Barbara ten days later telling us how much easier it was to express her emotions. She was crying more and feeling very good about it. Her friends had previously told her how worried they were about her because she seemed to keep her pain deep inside.

Barbara has needed four doses of the *Kali bromatum* over the year and a half we have treated her, in addition to taking lower

doses infrequently when she felt it was necessary. She has benefited tremendously from homeopathy — as has her son Ben —
and she has not needed to resume taking Zoloft.

"I Lost the Love of My Life"

Terry, a thirty-year-old part-time receptionist from Eastern
Washington, had a sadness about her. This was with good reason. Five years earlier, her husband, an experienced firefighter,
had perished while trying to rescue a family from their burning home. Since his death, Terry suffered from recurrent, often
drastic, mood swings. Her daughter was only three months old
when her husband died, and her son four years old. She and her
husband had been best friends.

Terry had visited the house where her husband perished. Due
to the circumstances, she wasn't able to identify her husband's
body for three days. It was a terrible shock that he had been so
disfigured by the fire that his body was unrecognizable. Terry
didn't cry immediately. She was so stunned, as if it were unreal
or a bad movie. At first it was like it did not even happen. Terry
would keep looking for her husband to come home. "I just
wanted to get away from everyone and everything. I wanted to
hide." She would have slept all day and all night if she hadn't had
to take care of her children. Then she experienced a period of
being unable to sleep at all.

Initially Terry and the kids stayed with her parents. It was when
they moved out and found a new place for themselves that the
gravity of the situation set in. It was odd, she thought, that she
didn't cry more after her husband's death. "When I started
crying, it would be over in a couple of minutes. It would just
shut off. I tended to keep my feelings to myself because I didn't
think people wanted to hear about it." Six months of counseling
helped a bit. Terry tried a couple of antidepressants but quit
because they made her feel dull and lifeless.

When Terry first came to see us, she still thought about her
husband all the time. She continually asked herself why he had

to die when he was such a good person. Terry became plagued by fears of something bad happening to her children. The periods of crying were now occasional and brief. Her mood was either really good or she would feel terrible about herself and the world around her, triggered by something insignificant.

Friends confided that they did not know what to expect from one minute to the next. Aware that she needed to move on with her life, Terry just couldn't get past the grief. Her desire to have another close relationship was eclipsed by her fear that if she loved someone again, something terrible might happen to that person, too.

Despite the fact that she was an excellent mother, Terry worried that she was not raising her children right and that they would suffer from not having a father. She made every effort to "keep it together" so that the kids would not be affected by her pain. They, in turn, were preoccupied about their mom and gave her lots of hugs and kisses to make her feel better.

One recurrent dream came to Terry many times: Her husband was not really dead, but she could see him only now and then. At first he would hug her and assure her that everything was okay. The last time that Terry had that dream, it felt as though he no longer wanted her.

Following her husband's death, a very disturbing tightness had developed and persisted in her throat and chest, often spreading to her stomach, arms and legs. She experienced periodic headaches and a knotted feeling in her stomach. The left side of her body felt weak, almost numb, so she preferred to sleep on her right side. Terry's hair came out in clumps and her weight fluctuated considerably. Even five years after the accident, Terry still had no real appetite for anything. Whatever she put into her mouth made her feel sick. She seemed to have lost her taste for fruit, juice and sweets, and when she did eat, she preferred spicy food.

We gave Terry a single dose of *Ignatia* (St. Ignatius bean), an excellent medicine for acute or chronic grief. Following that

87

dose she had a brief positive response, then again felt unfocused and hopeless. We knew that Terry fitted the picture of *Ignatia* and wondered whether anything could have interfered with the treatment. She told us she had been using Bag Balm and coffee regularly, two substances that can sometimes prevent homeopathic medicines from continuing to act. We instructed Terry to discontinue these products and repeat the dose of *Ignatia*.

Three months after her initial visit, Terry looked bright and cheerful. "I feel much better. No more mood swings. I'm pretty leveled out. Just feeling good. Little things don't bother me anymore. I can go with the flow. I feel more settled. The hopeless feelings are gone." She felt well even though her husband's birthday — an event that would have previously sent Terry into a tailspin — had just passed. Under stressful situations, the tightness in the chest recurred slightly, but it was no longer overwhelming and paralyzing. Her headaches were 70% better. The knots in the stomach were gone, as was her left-sided numbness. The concerns about something bad happening to her children were no longer present and friends no longer expressed concern about her mood swings. Terry was now buying tubs of fruit and no longer had such a desire for spicy food. She has continued to feel well and has not needed further treatment.

This is a typical response to homeopathic treatment for grief. When Judyth was a psychiatric social worker in the emergency room of a busy city hospital, part of her job was to console families whose relatives had died in the emergency room. In addition to whatever soothing words were appropriate, the families were offered Valium to assuage their grief. What a difference it could make for people in this type of situation if homeopathic medicines were available.

"My Husband Left Me and I Can't Go On"

Dorothy was a successful fifty-year-old architect from the Bay Area who had been treated with homeopathy for ten years. Her original complaint was poor digestion with frequent bloating and belching. Dorothy was self-conscious about being married to a man fifteen years younger than her. Premature graying of her hair contributed to her concerns about being old and undesirable, although she was quite an attractive woman. She had received benefit over the years from several homeopathic medicines, especially *Lycopodium* (club moss) and *Ignatia*. Then we didn't see Dorothy for a number of years because she was doing well.

Dorothy returned in great distress after her husband had recently moved out, having confessed ambivalence about staying in the marriage. Crazy about him, Dorothy experienced terrific despair. It seemed to her that the decision to divorce or remain together was in her husband's hands and that she was helpless to influence his decision. Dorothy explained, "The state of my marriage affects everything. It's an issue of self-esteem. Homeopathy has helped me in the past with stress and now I need help more than ever. I'm desperately unhappy. I contemplated suicide. I cry so easily. I don't know why. Maybe it's the menopause, maybe the marriage. It represents a loss of my femininity. I'm not sleeping well lately. I have so much on my mind. I don't know what to do with my life. I don't want to be rejected." Dorothy knew about rejection. Her childhood was difficult. An abusive marriage followed. She felt guilty about not having shown her children as much love as she would have liked due to her own emotional pain.

Dorothy's physical complaints included uterine fibroids, irregular periods, a nodular thyroid diagnosed as Hashimoto's thyroiditis and a tingling sensation from the neck upward. She loved carbo-hydrates, including rice, pasta and bread. Dorothy remarked that she had never been a thirsty person.

We prescribed *Ignatia*, which had helped Dorothy in the past, without success. Her condition had deteriorated. She was now tormented by thoughts of suicide, mainly of slitting her wrists. She felt no optimism about a future without her husband. She knew she would not kill herself, yet the urge to cut herself with a knife was persistent and disturbing.

89

When we probed further, Dorothy explained that she had a very domineering mother who allowed her to have absolutely no privacy. She was not encouraged to be herself. Her mother had picked out all of Dorothy's clothes, even in college. Dorothy only went out with boys that her parents liked. Her husband had become everything to her — the only person she ever loved and trusted.

Alumina (aluminum), a medicine for individuals who do not develop a healthy sense of self or individual identity, generally due to a rigid upbringing, was prescribed. Many people go through life borrowing ideas, beliefs and preferences of others since they have not acquired their own. They can become quite dependent on others, as in Dorothy's case. Knowing that people needing this medicine often suffer from longstanding constipation, we had inquired about Dorothy's bowel patterns and discovered constipation had been a significant problem throughout her childhood.

Dorothy called two weeks later and reported, "There's definitely been a major change. It's quite miraculous. I feel in so many ways back to myself. I hardly think of my husband. I've started being interested in other men again. People can see the change in me." Her physical symptoms were also diminished.

Over the next six months, the improvement continued. "I feel much more in touch with myself, like who I was before. I feel like I'm starting a new life. I've gone through some periods of depression, but I can stand outside of it and look at it. I can go into dark places, observe them, and come out quickly. I'm surprised at how resilient I feel. I talked to my husband. I didn't have any strong feelings about him. You reach a point where you can't overreact to all of it." She had no more urges to cut her wrists. Three months after taking the medicine, her medical doctor found no more nodules on her thyroid.

Dorothy needed six doses of *Alumina* over the next three years, during which she developed a much stronger sense of self. Previously she had looked to others to establish that sense. This was no longer necessary. She felt more sexual, attractive and hopeful. She has expressed a strong desire to connect with a man in an enduring relationship but in a more whole and healthy way than before the *Alumina*. Although her moods fluctuate somewhat, she generally is quite healthy and she has no desire whatsoever to be with her ex-husband, who has since remarried. Dorothy has been a homeopathic patient for sixteen years and relies on it as her primary source of health care, consulting conventional medical doctors infrequently.

13 I've Been Depressed Forever

Overcoming Lifelong Depression

There are some people who seem to come out of the womb sad. One or both parents may have suffered from depression or another mental illness. They may have been drug or alcohol abusers. Perhaps the circumstances of the pregnancy and birth were less than ideal, or even tragic, such as when the father of the child, or another loved one, dies during the pregnancy. Or, as is too often the case, the baby is unwanted, neglected or mistreated by one or both parents. There are many reasons a child may be depressed from the very beginning of life. This is a tough way to come into the world.

"I Felt Broken ... a Failure"

Angie, a thirty-two-year-old artist with curly brown hair and lots of freckles, was referred to us by her psychotherapist due to longstanding depression. "It's been a hard year," she confided. "I feel frustrated and stuck — like I've failed. It's mostly the eating and the depression. I've had problems with food since I was ten years old. I've been on so many diets. I've lost sixty pounds at a time, but then I just gained it all back. At other times I just stopped worrying about what I ate and tried to be gentle and forgiving with myself.

"I've gone to many therapists and sometimes it's been helpful. But I wonder if I'm doing therapy well enough, working hard enough at it. Am I doing it right? Last year everything kind of fell apart. Now I'm feeling very hopeless. I just don't see myself changing or getting better. I'm not finding the peace that I want.

"I know eating is just a symptom of a deeper issue. I tried to kill myself earlier this year. They put me in the hospital twice. Part of me has just given up trying. I get so stuck. I can't seem to get these negative messages out of my head: that I can't do anything right, that I'm not as good as others think, that I could disappear and it would be okay."

Angie had been quite matter-of-factly suicidal. Believing that she was wasting her time and that of her friends, and running out of ideas about what to try next to relieve her hopelessness, she took antidepressants along with alcohol. Angie was quite serious about ending her life. Her suicide attempt landed her in the local emergency room, then a psychiatric ward. When discharged and taking Wellbutrin, she remained depressed but functional.

Friends were the center of Angie's life. She referred to herself as "the tireless, thankless giver". She was there for her friends and they for her. She considered herself a passionate explorer of life. Yet she was continually disturbed by the belief that she was not the fabulous, capable person that others thought her to be.

Angie's inability to take control over her eating symbolized to her that she couldn't do anything right. She had begun to sneak food when she was ten, which had escalated to serious bingeing in high school and college. Angie could down an entire cake at a sitting.

A high achiever, Angie was the offspring of two professors. Her father took his own life while suffering from leukemia. Angie was proud of the way her father ended his life. She questioned whether she had a purpose for continuing to live. Her physical problems were few, consisting of some warts on her heels and dandruff. She had her gall bladder removed in her mid-twenties.

A single dose of homeopathic *Aurum metallicum* dramatically turned Angie's life around. At her five-week follow-up visit, she reported having more energy and not being as scared of life. She experienced little mood "dips" but no feelings of hopelessness. Her bingeing had stopped, although she was afraid to talk about it in case that might jinx her progress. Angie's thinking was considerably better. The negative, self-reproaching voice inside of her was less audible. She was impressed by the noticeable change in herself.

Two months later, Angie came in and reported feeling great. Her mind was extremely clear. She no longer felt hopeless, powerless and stuck. She was still taking Trazadone and Wellbutrin but felt substantially better than when she was only taking the drugs prior to homeopathic treatment. Even though she was a tremendous support to her friends, Angie was reluctant to ask anyone for help when she was hurting. Concerned about her state of mind, we called her eleven months later to see how she was doing. Angie reluctantly came back to see us and admitted that she had relapsed several months earlier. We gave her another dose of *Aurum* but the same positive response did not occur.

Interviewed further, Angie spoke at length about sadness and friends. Her greatest fear was being left, expendable, not needed. If she felt excluded or disappointed by those close to her, Angie retreated and erected a protective wall between herself and them. A vulnerable, creative, artistic woman, Angie was exquisitely sensitive to having her feelings hurt. Escapes for her included reading almost anything she could get her hands on, watching movies and eating — her foods of choice being cheese, rich or salty foods and ice cream. When we asked how Angie felt about music, she shared that she used music to stimulate a catharsis. If she felt blue, she played sentimental, emotional music, which made her even more melancholic until she was able to release her feelings.

This additional information led to a different prescription: *Natrum muriaticum* (sodium chloride). At her appointment six weeks later, Angie shared that her moods were much more stable. More energetic and focused, she was able to stay level emotionally even during the holidays, which had been impossible previously. She was no longer so sensitive to having her feelings hurt and the desire to binge was gone. Angie felt more involved with life and the need to escape into television or movies was less.

Angie reported after two more months that she felt fine. She would have been a candidate for long-term homeopathic treatment but has not continued under our care. We hear from another patient that now, several years later, she continues to function well.

Aurum metallicum is well suited to people who demand a great deal of themselves and are not satisfied with their performance, which can lead to severe, even suicidal, depression. Those needing *Natrum muriaticum* are generally very focused on friendships and one-on-one relationships. When they feel rejected, disappointed or abandoned, the loneliness and grief can be extremely profound.

"I Had No Communication with My Mother"

Anastasia, fifty-six years old, emigrated from Russia with her husband, Igor, in 1965. We began to see her in 1984, but she came in for care only sporadically for acute problems such as sciatica. We were able to delve into her problems more in depth when she came in very uncomfortable due to menopausal symptoms. "I was given estrogen even though I was still having periods, but I stopped after I read it could cause cancer. The doctor also prescribed diuretics because my blood pressure was high, but I didn't take them because they destroy the kidneys and I had kidney problems years ago. After all, I believe in natural medicine.

"I have lots of aches and pains. My feet are hot and burning, my right shoulder muscles are weak and painful, my eyelids swell, and my sciatica on the right side causes me to feel needles in the bottom of my right foot. My hands tremble, I'm tired all the time, and I can't sleep more than two to three hours at a time. All I want to eat is sweets, bread and salt. And I'm having nightmares about dead people who want to kill me or about thieves breaking into the house and I have to struggle to keep them out. I cry or scream, sometimes waking the rest of the family, but it's not even my voice.

"I was born in St. Petersburg. We were fifteen children, all with the same father and different mothers. My father had lots of women. We lived with my father and stepmother because my mother left when I was nine. My father was strict and I had almost no communication with my mother; I feel empty when I look at their pictures. It makes me feel sad that my mother

95

had such an unhappy life of silent suffering. I love my own children but I haven't been real affectionate with them. I never had a mother so I never knew how to be a mother.

"When my mother left, I prayed that I might be taken to heaven so I wouldn't have to live with my stepmother. She did not love me at all. My father had money, so they sent me to boarding school; but my sisters stayed at home. I was only allowed to go home over the weekends. My stepmother found reason to criticize me no matter what I did. I couldn't do anything right. She insisted on apologies but I refused. When my father punished us, we could be in our rooms for a week. He beat me for not helping my stepmother more. Once, when I was seventeen, I held my father's gun to my head but there was no bullet.

"I never had real friends. Father wouldn't allow it. At nineteen I left home with my sister, but my mother came to get us. I went to work, but she made me give all the money to her. Life was no better than before. My boyfriend, Igor, wanted to marry me. I didn't really love him but I had to get out of the house, so I agreed. We eventually moved to the United States and had our children. Igor went out with other women and never wanted to work, so I supported the family doing housecleaning. Five years ago he went back to Russia without telling me and I haven't heard from him since. A couple of years ago I married a wonderful man. I still clean in order to supplement his income. If there's a problem, I smile. My son says I want everything to be tranquil in order to avoid conflict. I work hard and I give to others."

Anastasia fit the picture of *Natrum muriaticum*: a sensitive, refined person who grieves internally (just as Anastasia's mother did) and feels tremendous disappointment and rejection. There is often a history of a lack of nurturing, of distance or difficulties in the relationship with one's mother. The desire for salt and bread are also typical.

When Anastasia came back to see us seven weeks later, she felt much better. The sciatica, burning of her feet, eye swelling and trembling were all gone. Her blood pressure was normal. She no longer dreamed of dead people or robbers and felt much more at peace. That was three years ago and Anastasia has not needed further homeopathic treatment. Homeopathy cannot change the family into which we were born and the circumstances of our childhoods. It can, however, help us to heal our past hurts and make a dramatic difference in how we respond to our lives in the present.

"I Never Felt She Was My Mother or I Was Her Daughter"

Edith, a sixty-five-year-old financial planner in Minnesota, first consulted us for depression and fatigue four years ago. "My family-practice doctor told me that you could help me. I came down with chronic fatigue syndrome two years ago. I got the flu and within ten days my knees buckled and I couldn't hold up my head. It took a year before my energy felt normal. Two months ago I got a virus, which triggered the symptoms again. It's strange that I got another flu because I went for a flu shot last fall.

"I have some close friends, but I'm fairly reclusive and introverted. There's no support from my immediate family. Not having a partner or family leaves a hole in my life. I'm hooked on cigarettes. A fifty-year smoker. Addictions have been my way to try to fill the empty place inside of me. When I inhale, I'm taking something into myself. I've tried everything to stop, but part of me doesn't want to let go of it. I just want to smoke to kill myself, but I don't want to get emphysema in the meantime. You are my last chance for help.

"My childhood was horrendous. My mother got pregnant at sixteen, then married someone else — not my father. She never wanted me. When I was twenty she told me she'd tried to abort me with a clothes hanger. I almost starved to death a week after my birth because my mother's nipples were inverted and they couldn't find a formula that I could keep down. I've been starving ever since.

"I don't ever recall my mother touching me as a child. She never protected me. I never felt she was my mother or I was her daughter. I was left at all-night movies when I was six. They would lock me in the car, then go to the bar and drink all night. I've blocked out most of my childhood because it was so awful.

"I didn't belong anywhere. In high school I came close to being catatonic. Very withdrawn. I've had a lot of therapy but I've sustained some really traumatic things [from] when I was very young, which set the pattern of being a loner, of living defensively. I started out with ten strikes against me, and I've spent my whole life pulling myself up. I've been married twice. I really wasn't capable of picking the right partner. My one son was quite willful and difficult from day one. We've had a certain amount of conflict between us in the past, and we aren't close now.

"My depression was terrible when I got the chronic fatigue. It's as if someone put a black bag over my head. I was suicidal. Even though I'm dead set against drugs, I went on Imipramine for two months, then I got over it. Now that I'm feeling tired again, the depression is returning. I'd call it a despair. Like everything's going downhill. Nothing will fix my life. I'm a very sensitive and compassionate person, and I can't stand to hear about others' pain and suffering. Crowds are hard for me. I'm uncomfortable around people I don't know. Probably because I was isolated all the time growing up. I don't feel lonely because I have my furry friends: a kitty and a collie."

Edith never felt rested. She woke up just as tired as when she went to bed. Her eyes were chronically puffy, she complained of urinary dribbling and incontinence, and she had a lifelong aversion to eating. Recently Edith noticed that when she bent forward, she felt as if her heart were in a vise. If she sat at her desk with clients for long periods of time, she felt pain around her heart. She had a history of infrequent transient ischemic attacks.

Fortunately we were able to help Edith with *Aurum metallicum*, quite beneficial for sufferers of deep — even suicidal — depression, especially in combination with heart problems. Five weeks after taking the *Aurum*, Edith told us, "I am so good. Better than I've felt in many months. I had quite a fast, dramatic response to the medicine. My heart problem has stabilized. I consulted a cardiologist and was diagnosed with a right-bundle branch block. I've been feeling very positive. I've cut down to a pack of cigarettes every week or two. My son is coming for a visit and I feel real comfortable about it. I'm in a much better place than I've been in a long time."

Now sixty-nine, Edith has done quite well since beginning the *Aurum*. She has needed periodic doses over the past four years, often due to dental work, but has continued to feel much, much better than before beginning homeopathic treatment. She has stopped smoking, her heart condition continues to be stable and her outlook on life has improved considerably.

14 Life Is Just Too Much to Handle!

Lightening the Load of a Hectic Life

We live in a busy, fast-paced, complex society — bearing the responsibilities of family, home and job. The simple life of the '40s and '50s is gone. Our highly technological world has led to more choices and decisions, often split-second. Paying the bills, keeping up with phone calls, beeper calls, faxes and e-mail. Living from paycheck to paycheck. Or, for some, having so much money that they don't know how to spend it. We are struck by how stressful the lives of children are today. Often gone from morning till night, carrying beepers so they won't miss out on anything, playing video games as fast as possible. They barely have time to grow up! Too much work, too little enjoyment and not enough heartfelt connection with other people. This is a prescription for unhappiness.

"A Half-Empty Kind of Guy"

Max, forty, was burned out. A telephone-cable repair supervisor from St. Louis, he was just plain exhausted, not to mention discouraged with his life and his job requiring long hours on the road. He described himself as a simple, down-to-earth man in a hustle-bustle world. Bored and overwhelmed with his job of twelve years, he also felt distant from his girlfriend. Stress at work and more stress at home. It just felt like too much. Max told us he felt like there were "two hammers beating on me at the same time".

A great hindsight critic, Max had a litany inside his head about what he could have or should have done differently. A constant second-guesser when it came to all of his perceived mistakes, he complained of below-average self-esteem. Bombarded with decision making, he based his choices on fear rather than intuition. Filled with self-doubt, he never felt he had enough on the ball to succeed in his undertakings. This led Max to have an "I'd better take what I can get" philosophy about his possibilities and capabilities. Although he had begun to interview for another job, he never felt he had a ghost of a chance of being hired elsewhere. The truth was that Max's employers placed a lot of value on his expertise, but he never believed it. He described himself as a "half-empty kind of guy".

The product of a typical Midwestern farm family, Max felt unjustly punished by his father. "I got the message that I couldn't do anything right, and it stuck with me." Like glue. Max's feelings about his life were those of total loss, failure and helplessness. When he felt worst, he was gripped by a tight feeling in his chest and a loss of appetite. Rather than look at what he could change in his environment or what role others played in his disappointments, Max pointed the finger at himself, just as his father had done to him. His inner dialogue went like this: "What can I do to improve myself? I thought I was trying, but I guess I'm not doing it well enough."

Ultimately Max felt quite desperate and anxious, as well as clueless about how to remedy his life. He called himself a defeatist but could not figure out how to pull himself out of the pit. He lamented, "I've failed in so many ways, made so many stupid decisions in my life. I mull things over to death, afraid of making the wrong decision. Everyone is dissatisfied with me. It's too much to bear." When we asked what was unusual about him, he answered, "I'm a nobody. I know that's a pretty sad statement but that's how I feel. Wrung through the wringer."

Max had never done well in school, mostly Cs, Ds and Fs, even though he was an intelligent man. Convinced that he would fail, he panicked before tests and inevitably was the last to finish. Awkward in social situations, he didn't speak unless he was very sure. "I go off and sit by myself or dismiss myself. I don't fit." Max's greatest fear was of negativity, even though he knew he generated it himself. "I don't trust the human world. I feel like a pea in the ocean and there's nothing to do about it." Max dreamed about unfinished projects.

The first medicine we gave Max, *Aurum metallicum*, had little effect. However, he benefited considerably from *Cadmium sulphuricum*, a medicine for depressed, discouraged individuals who feel stuck and unable to move. Though their ideals may be high and they may be quite capable, they never feel that way. Their performance anxiety is great because they suffer from such tremendous self-doubt and reproach. This metal is actually used in telephone cables, so it is interesting that Max, who worked with the cables for many years, needed this particular substance. Perhaps his state was brought on by the continual exposure to the substance.

Six weeks after taking the *Cadmium sulphuricum,* Max felt less desperate. Whereas he acknowledged feeling "beside himself" prior to the homeopathy, now he enjoyed more periods of being at ease. "I'm not so focused on the problems at hand. I feel more able to come up with a solution. I've seen some possibilities to get out of my situation. My outlook is moving forward."

Over the next six and a half months Max continued to improve. He actually changed jobs and his spirits improved. He and his girlfriend were getting along better. "I'm not at all depressed. I'm actually pleasantly surprised when I step outside myself and look in." Seven months after the original dose of the *Cadmium sulphuricum,* Max felt that he was slipping when lots of pressure came up in his new job. The self-blame had begun to creep back. We repeated the medicine at that time.

Many people believe that once a failure, always a failure. This case shows that, with the right kind of help, that is not necessarily true.

"I Felt God Calling Me"

Meg, a forty-year-old clothing designer, was the middle child of three children. She first came to see us four years ago, and we have subsequently treated her two daughters and her mother as well. Although Meg was quite close to her mom, her father was a mean, critical and abusive alcoholic. Meg's grandfather made sexually suggestive advances toward her, which caused her to lose her trust in him. Meg's family moved from California to Florida when she was twelve. Not only was she traumatized by moving far away from all of her friends, but, to make matters worse, her father followed in her grandfather's footsteps. When she rejected her father's advances, he decided to just ignore her. So not only did she lose her grandfather, but she lost her father as well. Meg's father was cruel and vicious toward her mother, so Meg was too afraid for her mother's safety to tell her what happened. She kept it all to herself.

"What I did in response to all of these traumas was to take care of my little brother, to protect him. Rejected and betrayed by the girls at school, I felt isolated, out of the loop."

Meg found another outlet for her pent-up secret: compulsive eating. Her saving grace was that at this time God came into her life. "I felt God calling me. It's the one thing in my life that is surefire." Having faced disappointment and rejection, Meg vowed to make sure everyone liked her. God served as a faithful companion, even when Meg was mortified after her dad showed up drunk at her high school graduation. "Listening to God, talking to God. He leads me out of isolation into wholeness."

Meg met her future husband while she was in college majoring in fashion. He was in law school. "Shortly after I met him, an angel told me we'd marry. It's been difficult because he's such a fearful person. I want to be a good wife but my feelings are often frozen. We have two little girls and really want to work things out. My husband is a successful lawyer and provides quite well for us. I know how much he loves me. He's just afraid of life.

"I feel sad about all the trauma in my life. Very sorrowful. I used to feel such passion, and now sorrow cuts at the very root of it." Meg dreamed of being in prison. "First I was in prison with my father and now in my marriage." She also had dreams of her sorrow melting like ice and of finding her way to happiness. A devoted wife and mother, Meg felt very responsible for the happiness of her family. Yet she felt trapped, as her dreams revealed. Meg had only one friend with whom she could share her deepest feelings. She wouldn't think of tarnishing the reputation of her husband, a prominent lawyer with political aspirations.

Abdominal complaints had troubled Meg for the previous five years. The cramps came during moments of being alone with her husband or getting in touch with her grief. Her emotional pain wore on Meg. The only thing that relieved her fatigue was chocolate. In moments of despair, she would eat a couple of handfuls of Hershey's kisses between sobs. In addition to chocolate, Meg loved butter, rich ice cream and cream cheese. She also suffered from occasional headaches, mostly when she spent time with her husband.

It took some time to find the medicine that helped Meg most dramatically. During the first year of treatment, she derived some benefit from *Sepia* (cuttlefish ink) and homeopathic *Chocolate*, but without a doubt the most profound change came after giving her *Natrum carbonicum* (sodium carbonate). This medicine is for very sensitive people who feel a profound sense of isolation. Refined and very willing to help and serve others, they often carry inside a deep sense of emptiness and separation. They commonly suffer from gas and bloating, as did Meg.

Three weeks after taking the *Natrum carbonicum*, the abdominal cramps and fatigue were gone. Her chocolate craving evaporated, and her tendency to overeat disappeared for the first time in twenty-five years. "I've begun to feel a love for myself that I've never felt before. My dreams are very positive. My feelings don't get hurt so easily. I realize that my husband and I are separate people and that our journeys are different and that's good. I used to have a foggy feeling in my head. That's pretty much gone." After another three weeks Meg reported, "I'm out of the pit. Every single problem that I've talked to you about has improved after taking this medicine."

Six months after we switched medicines for Meg, she shared with us more about her long history of feeling isolated from friends. "My main stance with people has been 'Please don't dislike me. You can leave me alone, but please don't exclude me.' I was my mom's best friend. She had the habit of saying

I didn't need other friends because I had her. My mom considered me her confidante and she never liked my friends. I made a kind of inner vow of acceptance that I couldn't have other friends, that my mom and friends didn't mix. Any other friend would be an intrusion on my relationship with my mother. The other night I woke up and realized this so clearly. You know, I asked for a dream about friends and this is my answer."

During the three years since beginning the *Natrum carbonicum*, we have seen Meg much less frequently for treatment and she has needed only one repetition of the medicine, which was over one year ago. She is much better adjusted in her marriage and derives greater enjoyment than ever from spending time with her family and friends.

"I Never Got Any Advice from My Parents"

Melanie, a thirty-five-year-old mom, came to see us for chronic sinus problems and to improve her overall health. She felt overwhelmed by the responsibility of raising two sons. Her husband, an insurance salesman, traveled all over the Northwest. They had moved to Seattle from Portland two years earlier. Melanie wept as she told us, "I haven't connected to many people here. I used to have really close friends that I could trust. I could tell them anything, even call them at two in the morning for help. I just don't feel that sense of safety with any of my friends here. It makes me feel very lonesome.

"What I miss the most is bouncing my ideas off of my friends and having different perspectives to consider. Here I have to do it all myself. I'm proud of my teaching and my mothering but I still feel scared and alone. Scared of not making the right choices for my students and my family — of not knowing enough. I really miss talking to someone, giving that person my thoughts and ideas and then having that person help me sift through them and focus. That process makes me feel confident. Other people give me more ideas and solutions and help me realize things aren't such a problem after all.

"For example, I wasn't very happy with my children's pediatrician but I wasn't sure what to do about it. I talked to another mother who raved about her children's doctor. That helped me make the decision to switch. I feel very proud of my decisions, but I can feel split while I am trying to decide. I see both sides of everything so it can be pretty confusing. I miss the support and encouragement that I used to get from my girlfriends in Portland.

"I think I've felt this way forever. I was a happy kid, so my parents pretty much left me alone. My parents focused more on my gifted sister and my older brother who had lots of emotional problems." When we asked Melanie if she got much advice from her parents, her eyes started to tear up. "No. They just echoed what I said. They never told me whether my ideas were good or bad or offered another alternative. Sometimes I really wanted advice but I never got any. Like when it came to choosing colleges. My gifted sister went to one of the best colleges in the country. My parents just asked me where I was applying and told me, 'Whatever you want,' but they never helped me decide which school to choose."

Melanie had dreams of being in the delivery room helping out a friend during labor. She felt happy that she was able to help her friend.

It was clear to us that Melanie sought guidance and help. Having left her close friends behind in Portland, she felt lonely and unsupported, even though she had an excellent relationship with her husband. This was a case for *Strontium carbonicum* (strontium carbonate). Six weeks after taking the medicine, Melanie's sinus complaints had improved by 70 to 80%. She felt much calmer and more centered and no longer experienced a sense of being split.

It has now been over a year since she first came to see us and she has needed infrequent doses of the *Strontium carbonicum*. She is more able to do things by herself. She is much more able to stand up for what she wants and to handle the challenges of everyday life without feeling overwhelmed. She is sleeping more deeply and has made several new friends, which has made her quite happy.

"My Stomach Is Tied in Knots"

Audrey, a fifty-nine-year-old, was a fashion retailer from Spokane. Desipramine had helped her temporarily with depression, but when she had stopped taking it she crashed again. Now, back on the medication, she sought another answer. "I cry easily and doubt my self-worth. I don't feel like I have anything to contribute to the world. My stomach is tied in knots.

"I've felt this way before. First ten years ago when I divorced my husband, then five years ago when my finances ran amok. My enthusiasm and zest for life have evaporated. I can't seem to hold things together. I'm not my usual happy, effervescent self. My family is a mess. My son was recently hospitalized for depression. My daughter and I aren't communicating well. My sister is dying from ovarian cancer. I have a constant churning in my stomach from anxiety.

"Depression runs in my family. I lost my parents in my midtwenties. They died within six months of each other. I was devastated. First my father died suddenly of an aneurysm, then my mother died of a broken heart. Being the oldest of six, I felt responsible for my siblings. Not knowing what to do, I was filled with feelings of inadequacy. My first husband was an alcoholic and we divorced. Somehow I found ways to cope because I knew it was necessary, that is until recently.

"Ten years ago I finally fell apart. The realization of how inadequate I was to be in this world. My job performance suffered. I guess the feeling that best describes it is despair. Feeling lost, not knowing what to do. I've been a supporter, a pleaser. Now, for the first time, I'm thinking about myself. I'm tired of being responsible. I want to retire, travel, spend time with my grandchildren. My ambition is gone. I don't feel I've done a great job raising my family, and I've never been as successful in sales as I would have liked. I felt guilty about not spending enough time with the kids because of my work and for neglecting my work for the kids. Once, I opened my own fabric store but it went bankrupt. Everyone knew that I'd failed. My marriage was also failing at the time. I feel like I've failed in life. I wonder what I could have done differently to make things work out better.

"There's nothing I've ever excelled at doing. Not from lack of conscientiousness. I reproach myself for doing the wrong thing. There's a continual pressure on me to perform. School was never easy for me. I transpose letters. Remembering numbers or memorizing information has been a challenge. It's hard to retain what I've read. I was overweight for years and used to be very self-conscious. I worked hard to lose weight and become attractive again, and I get irritated with people like my son who don't take care of themselves.

"Everyone in my family was a dentist, so I have a mouth full of gold. Lots of fillings and a couple of root canals. I had acne as a young adult and took tons of antibiotics."

We gave Audrey a single dose of *Aurum metallicum* (gold), a good medicine for depressed individuals who carry the burdens of others on their shoulders, have very high standards of performance and rarely feel up to the task at hand. It may or may not be a coincidence that Audrey's mouth was filled with gold.

When we next saw Audrey, two months later, she told us she felt great. "I don't cry anymore. I'm happy and don't feel overwhelmed. In fact I feel at peace. My life is much more in control. The change has been gradual. My psychiatrist has reduced my Desipramine to 25 milligrams a day, and I have told her that my intention is to gently go off of it. I felt fine during the holidays. I've decided to leave my job selling clothing and market greeting cards instead."

Four months later Audrey still felt quite well. "A lot calmer. Not as agitated. Clearer mind. Much more balanced. It's just delightful to feel so much better. I gave up selling cards because it wasn't fun, and I retired. I stay busy around the house. Spending more time with my grandchildren is a joy. I am in a very compatible relationship and we're planning to get married. I've had more gas but I'm not too worried about it. There are several fillings that I need to have replaced over the next month or so."

Audrey needed one repetition of the *Aurum* following the dental work and a second after she felt worse after eating coffee ice cream. After one year of treatment, she is again feeling on top of things.

15 Alone on a Distant Island
Reconnecting with the Human Race

Ours is a lonely society: alarmingly high divorce rates, single-parent families, alienation among generations and races. Due to job relocations, divorce, necessity and preference, parent and child may live two to three thousand miles away from each other. In our ever more fast-paced and plastic society, many question what has happened to human and family values. Love and connection are fundamental human needs that are too often lacking. When a child misses the nurturing, bonding and support for which she yearns while growing up, she may never fully recover. Far too many lonely children grow into lonely adults, searching futilely for the love and affection they never received and may never be able to give.

"I'd Do Anything to Please"

Leanne, a twenty-eight-year-old receptionist from Olympia, was soft-spoken and extremely sweet. "I've been feeling a loss of self-esteem because of my weight. I go to school full-time and work part-time. I'm majoring in accounting but it wasn't my first choice. I don't like my job. I don't eat right or exercise right. I'm not very assertive. It takes a lot of arm-twisting to get me to go to a party, then I just go off and sit in a corner. It takes me a long time to get comfortable with people. Friends tell me I'm an introvert.

"My parents divorced when I was in the second grade. Like most kids my age, I thought it was my fault. I chose to live with my dad in another state, and I left my sister, Kate, with my mom. For the past ten years Kate has refused to talk to me. We were very close. Every time I talk about her, I cry. I'm sorry. There are two half siblings. At times they feel like my children because they're so much younger. I was there to help my dad financially and to take care of the kids.

"I was married once. To a jerk who put me down. He never worked and I supported him. I've managed to remove anything which reminded me of him. I don't want to feel I'm still supporting a freeloader.

"Most of the time I'm unhappy — mostly with my weight. But no matter how much I've weighed I've still been unhappy. I wish I could be more assertive. If someone asks me to do something, I just jump and do it, then I get mad at myself. I guess I just want to feel needed. Pleasing my mom was the only way I made her happy. She was only happy with me when I was doing things for her. It hurt that mom didn't accept me, especially because it was so obvious that she loved my sister more than me. We were latchkey kids. I shared a bed with my mom. My sister had her own room. When I was thirteen, my sister and I decided to move out and live with my dad. While I was packing, I found out that my mother wouldn't let my sister come with me. It was very traumatic.

"My stepmother told me to lie about my half siblings so she and my father wouldn't have to send more money to my mother. I kept the secret for years. I'm resigned that my mother never loved me. My sister won't even talk to me. I feel very, very hurt. I keep trying to contact her but she won't talk to me. I feel like I want to go forward, but I don't know how. People say I'm fun but I don't see why.

"I would most like to learn to accept myself. I feel like other people see me as a wallflower. I typically get called by other people's names. I'd gained about seventy-five pounds around the time I moved out on my own and I'm still overweight. I mostly stay at home. All my books are there, so I'm safe. Nothing can happen there that I don't let happen. I'm happy that I'm not in an intimate relationship. Sometimes it's lonely, but I don't have to share my space with anybody."

A worrier by nature, Leanne feared big dogs, high places and losing weight. She didn't like to lose control. She was unwilling to go on walks or hikes by herself and was concerned that she might fail in school even though she was a good student. "I worry about anything, even whether the sky will turn blue." Leanne dreamed about being chased or driving too fast and the brakes failing, of a plane crashing, or about being a bug on a wall.

Her main physical complaint was tension headaches two or three times a month, which could last for days. Icy cold hands and feet also bothered her.

Leanne needed a medicine for gentle, soft-spoken, self-conscious individuals who are sensitive to criticism, are shy and fearful, and who have a strong need to please others. People who think they have to manage on their own without assistance and are prone to dreaming about accidents. We prescribed *Calcarea muriatica* (calcium chloride).

At her six-week visit Leanne reported feeling very well. "I feel like I'm standing on solid ground again. I'm more confident in myself, and I'm not worrying so much about what others are thinking or saying. I'm doing better in school and my grades are improving. I'm getting more A's. I can take more challenges. I wrote a letter to my ex-husband, telling him that I want the money he owes me now. I'm not getting depressed as often. I'm happy to say that I'm not letting people stomp all over me. Someone was being rude to me recently and I told her I didn't deserve to be treated that way. She went away, then came back and apologized for her rudeness. My fears are not so over-whelming. I can actually think of standing next to a cliff and not being worried. A dog came by and I didn't feel nervous.

"Homeopathy is wonderful. I've been sleeping so well that I don't want to wake up because I'm so relaxed. My feet and hands aren't cold anymore. I haven't had any anxiety dreams that wake me up. My headaches are really mild and less frequent. I still worry about things, but not to the same degree. As the foundation gets more solid, the worrying will go away. I just feel really, really good."

Leanne again, three months later: "I called my sister and told her when she was ready to have a sister that loved her uncondition-ally she could call me. I feel better overall. More centered and not as vulnerable to other people. The things I considered fright-ening before are challenges now." Leanne needed five doses of the *Calcarea muriatica* over a three-year period. We saw her last a year and a half ago and she has not needed further treatment.

"I Feel Excommunicated by My Family"

Ronny, forty years old, worked as a travel agent. Her early years had not been easy. She grew up in an Italian neighborhood in New York City. Ronny's grandparents came to this country from Milan. Her mother, at the age of thirty-two, had a third child. The baby died and Ronny's mother suffered a nervous breakdown. Ronny and her brother were sent to a Catholic orphanage. They thought they were responsible for the baby's death. Ronny cried herself to sleep every night that she was there.

After a time at home, Ronny and her brother were taken back to the orphanage by their father, an abusive and violent alcoholic. Living around her father had been a terrifying experience for Ronny. He beat her and her brother repeatedly. She hid in a garment bag, with a knife in case he found and attacked her when he came home from the bar drunk. There were times when she felt like she could have killed him. Ronny's mother also had a violent streak. She beat the kids with a frying pan, or whatever else she could get her hands on. Though Ronny often tried to protect her mother from her father's abuse, she basically felt betrayed by her.

Ronny and her brother eventually went back to live with their parents. When Ronny was fourteen, her parents finally divorced. Sent back to the orphanage once again, she received help from the nuns. At that time she had a revelation in the form of a visitation. She received instructions to speak the truth and not be afraid. After that she had the courage to stand up to her father.

At twenty-four, Ronny married her Italian boyfriend. Over time he became sexually abusive and slept with her sister. Her sister never spoke to her again. Jealous and resentful, Ronny left her husband, but he pursued her. She never felt vindicated for her betrayal by her husband and sister. The feeling she held toward her family was of rejection and excommunication. Ronny often felt attacked by her mother, her father, her husband and even by friends. Depression was a familiar companion and was even more pronounced when it rained. Ronny remarried and had a daughter but was tormented with fear that her ex-husband would kidnap her. She also feared heights and had a fascination with snakes. When she was little, she used to play with her brother's boa constrictor.

The resentment Ronny developed had taken hold in her stomach. Whenever she thought about her mother or about the betrayals, her "stomach would come out [her] mouth" and she would retch. She loved salads.

Ronny's intense feelings of jealousy, betrayal and resentment, and her need for vindication — in addition to her vomiting, aggravation from the rain and love of salads — led us to prescribe *Elaps* (coral snake). When we saw her two months later, she was quite pleased with her response to the medicine. Her attitude was much more positive. She felt more detached from her family and was no longer retching.

Two months later she reported that her feelings toward her family were much less intense despite a family dispute over her grandfather's estate after his recent death. She continued to feel well physically and was less afraid of heights. Two years after taking the *Elaps*, she continues to feel well and has not needed another dose of the medicine.

"My Life Is Barren"

Nancy, a social worker from New York, began her interview by telling us that she felt lonely, isolated, sad and overwhelmed. Forty-five years old, she realized that she was intelligent, strong and capable but was unable to find happiness. We had been able to help her son, who had attention deficit disorder, and she hoped we could help her turn around her life as well.

"I enjoy giving advice. I have caseload friendships. I'm there for them, but whenever I start to articulate my own needs, my friends leave. My work isn't fulfilling, I don't have a partner or anyone on the horizon. Most of my life is barren except for my spirituality. After spending two years in the Peace Corps in Africa, I fell in love with their native traditions and religion, and that is what I still practise. I find the connection with all of the creatures of nature — the music, the magic, the animal sacrifices — very satisfying. We have a community here, mostly African.

"I have a problem with men. My uncle abused me as a child, and I've had trouble ever since accepting men in authority. I recovered my memories of sexual abuse seven years ago and have not been sexually active since. For a long, long time I had an attachment to suicide. In major times of anguish, that's how I would comfort myself. I used to think about drowning or pills or driving off a cliff. Once I thought about shooting myself in my therapist's office. I was hospitalized for depression once. It's mainly the hopelessness about feeling like I'll never fill the emptiness. My son's life interferes with my being able to have a life.

"The pain comes from feeling that I can't fulfill my desires because I'm overweight and middle-aged. I don't have a lot of confidence in men as partners. What I'm really seeking is a spiritual connection. I've been married twice. My first marriage was emotionally barren for me, and the second was abusive. My money goes mainly for basics and for my son's needs. I want a cat but I can't find one I like. My twenty-year-old cat died a couple of years ago. She'd been with me throughout my adult life.

"If I try to become involved in others' lives or I try to deepen the relationships, I fail. So I convince myself that it's just going to keep happening that way. Such an emptiness. I've felt fragmented. A split: the life I've known about for forty-five years, and the life I found out about seven years ago. The incest started in infancy and continued until puberty. I remember being lonely and not wanting to be left alone. Actually I was completely alone from the very beginning. I never felt attached to anyone. Shy and isolated, I believed that my mother loved my sister more than me. I was smart and geeky and never had a lot of friends. My teachers perceived me as calm, quiet and nice. They sat me next to the problem kids so I'd have a good influence on them."

115

Nancy had numerous fears: of being alone for life, of revealing herself, of being hurt or rejected and of heights, as well as claustrophobia. She was terrified of being open to life, of allowing herself to experience joy because as soon as she felt it, someone might take it away from her. Nancy had one recurrent dream of surviving a huge tidal wave and another of narrowly escaping suffocation by an assailant. In a third dream, she was supposed to be taking care of a baby but didn't know how. She had still another dream about growling, snarling cats and dogs. Around the time she recovered her sexual-abuse memories, Nancy was tormented by nightmares.

A chocolate lover, Nancy in her childhood also sucked on lemons and ate salt out of her hand. She complained of frequent anxiety in her stomach and tightness in her throat, weak knees, dry lips, gas, insomnia, fatigue, stress, incontinence and an urge to urinate frequently, all day long.

Based on Nancy's profound feeling of isolation and disconnectedness, her strong attraction to animals, her distance from her son when he was an infant and even now feeling that he was restricting her freedom, and her craving for chocolate, we gave her homeopathic *Chocolate*. Nancy reported three months later that the medicine worked very well — almost immediately. "I started feeling fuller and less anxious pretty much right away. The feeling of a big hole was nearly gone. I stopped eating compulsively, started sleeping, the gas lessened, and I felt happier and more connected. The feeling of isolation left."

Nancy has continued to improve significantly. She experiences some periodic, mild feelings of isolation, but the emptiness never returned. For the first time in her life she feels like a grown-up adult. "I'm more capable of giving and receiving love. The feeling of isolation has changed texture. It's not so personal. My work is much more satisfying and I'm having lots of fun lately."

Nancy experienced a period of migraine headaches, which went away after a repetition of the same medicine. She also confided more about her pregnancy with her son. She had hated being pregnant because she felt nauseous the entire time. With absolutely no confidence that she knew what to do with a baby, she feared harming or losing him and kept herself at a distance. Nancy suffered from tremendous engorgement of her breasts while nursing, which was painful and unpleasant. We learned later that Nancy had been addicted to chocolate throughout her life. Her mom never let her buy candy bars, and one of the highlights of her college experience was having the freedom to buy Hershey's candy bars whenever she felt like it. We have found the ambivalence about being pregnant and mothering characteristic of women needing *Chocolate*.

Nancy has needed five doses of homeopathic *Chocolate* over the past two years. The profound emptiness and isolation never returned, her headaches are gone, she has very little gas, she sleeps well, she no longer complains about her job, and she is getting along very well with her son.

16 Worthless and Without Purpose

Rebuilding Self-Esteem and Confidence

A positive sense of self is an essential ingredient for happiness and success. Unfortunately, many people never develop the sense that they are of value and continue to hold the belief that no one else will value them either. This may result from being put down by parents or siblings, ridicule by peers, a recurrence of perceived failures in life and rejections or abandonment. Even though others may see the wonderful qualities of and possibilities for such a person, she remains stuck in self-reproach, the negative tapes playing over and over in her head. Some individuals have a tendency to undervalue themselves even though they are loved, cared for and respected. It's just a persistent lack of self-confidence that they can't shake. Although low self-esteem is not a condition that can necessarily change overnight, we have seen many patients turn around remarkably in terms of their ability to appreciate themselves, develop positive social relationships, and find happiness in their lives. The most powerful factors to inspire improvement in self-esteem are favorable changes in the quality of close relationships and work. (Andrews and Brown, p. 23) Once a person is able to break the barrier of her perceived limitations and find satisfying relationships, her entire life can turn around for the better.

Can one's self-esteem be too high? Although a poor self-image and self-reproach is far more common than a narcissistic personality, a new study by researchers at Iowa State University examined the type of inflated self-esteem that results from parents lavishing excessive, unwarranted praise on their children. They found that this type of unjustified self-aggrandizement can trigger hostility, aggression and violence. (Begley, p. 69) Like anything in life, happiness arises from the middle path — neither too much self-deprecation nor too much egotism.

The Measure of a Woman

Rachel worried incessantly — about her marriage, her finances and having her own business. Finances were tight and things were not going very well with her husband. Her anxiety showed up in her body as gas, heartburn and a nervous stomach.

The daughter of an alcoholic Montana farmer, Rachel, too, had an addictive nature. As a teenager she had used recreational drugs regularly. Now thirty, she had given up drugs and alcohol one year prior to consulting us for homeopathic treatment five years ago. A compulsive overeater, Rachel also had an addictive relationship with food. Her eating habits were erratic due to her rigorous schedule of working out. An athlete, she was a marathon runner, martial artist and aerobics teacher. She loved teaching aerobics. In fact, it was almost too exciting. "I get so keyed up and exhausted," she explained, "that I don't know who I am."

Getting up in front of people made Rachel edgy. In high school and college, she'd choose to fail a course rather than give an oral presentation. Now she faced the challenge of teaching forty students. She gave it everything she had "so others would not think she was chicken."

"I've been a worrier from day one," Rachel explained. "My parents divorced when I was five. My mother would cry all the time. First I lost my father, then when my brother was born, it was as if I lost my mother. I had no one. I became introverted and shy and would hardly talk at all. I was a tomboy and loved climbing trees. I was afraid of the dark, scary things and of being chased." At six, Rachel began to suffer from stomach aches and nightmares.

Her masculine side prevailed. "I'll take on any challenge to prove my worth. If other people think I'm all right, I must be okay. I'm very hard on myself." An experienced black-belt martial artist, Rachel had the skill to teach but lacked the confidence. Inside, Rachel felt a certain weakness that led her to want to mimic others. It was hard for her to open up and trust because she felt that she "might get squashed".

Rachel perceived sex as a form of domination. She just didn't trust her husband sexually. Attracted to women during the previous few years, she began to write sensual poetry about her fantasies and dreams.

The medicine that benefited Rachel tremendously is *Vanadium*. It is indicated for people who feel that they must perform at a very high level and be successful, but despite their capabilities they are filled with self-doubt. When they succeed they feel very good about themselves, but when they fail they are devastated and begin to question their self-worth. These individuals have a tendency toward eating disorders, such as anorexia and bulimia, the compulsive eating being a compensation for the lack of warmth and support. Digestive problems are often present.

Rachel described feeling much stronger, more solid and independent after taking the *Vanadium*. She no longer wanted to be with her husband, who was emotionally unavailable to her. She yearned to establish her own martial-arts school. Rachel felt less rigid about food. Three months later, Rachel reported that she had founded her martial arts school. She felt light and bubbly, and no longer felt compulsive about food. She developed venereal warts and decided to leave her husband. We repeated the medicine and her venereal warts disappeared.

Over the next year, Rachel divorced her husband, her martial arts school flourished, and she began a committed relationship with a woman that has made her very happy. Her confidence in herself and her abilities blossomed. During the past two years she has benefited from *Vanadium* for both acute illnesses and after two relapses of her chronic symptoms.

"I Never Feel Worthy"

Kelsey, a fifteen-year-old high school student, came in with her mom, a family-practice physician on the Olympic Peninsula. Her chief physical complaints were facial acne and fatigue.

"Sometimes I get depressed. A couple of nights ago I cried for an hour after I saw myself in a swimsuit. Any little thing can set me off. I hate to look in the mirror. I see the cellulite on my stomach; my hair's been falling out. I just can't live up to the form that our culture sees as perfect. Like the girls we see in magazines or on TV. I began to feel this way in the eighth grade when I started worrying how boys saw me. Or maybe even before the fifth grade when I went out with a boy and he made all of the other boys in the class hate me because my chest was flat. It was horrible. None of them would talk to me. I felt like I could never be worthy, that there would be something wrong with me — like I couldn't do anything right.

"I just feel insecure all the time. I worry about how others see me. That they're not seeing me the way I am on the inside. Often I wear baggy clothes so they won't see my unflattering parts. I have to hide my stomach. With all of my inhibitions, I can't have fun or be myself around boys. What if I say the wrong thing and they hate me again? It's like walking on eggshells. I had a relationship with a guy at my school last year. When he stopped seeing me, I blamed myself for not opening up enough to him. I tend to blame myself for everything that's wrong."

Her mom told us that Kelsey thought of herself as fat and ugly, even though she was quite attractive and by no means over-weight. An honor student, Kelsey was very hard on herself. She had a great fear of being misunderstood, of having people take her actions the wrong way. Kelsey agreed. "I do have pretty high standards for myself. I have a hard time appreciating my own efforts."

Kelsey also wanted help with what she called "cloudy thinking". Her only other complaints were a wart on her left foot and rest-less sleep. She loved garlic and hated onions.

This may sound like the typical story of a teenager growing up in America — acne, high self-expectations, caring too much what others think. But from a homeopathic point of view, some-thing was out of balance here. Kelsey was just too self-blaming, reacted too strongly to the boys turning against her in the fifth grade and was far too self-deprecating about her appearance. From the many patients we have seen with similar stories, we find it likely that if Kelsey's thoughts about herself continued in the same vein, she would have become anorexic or bulimic.

We gave Kelsey *Thuja* (tree of life), a medicine for people with low-self esteem who consider themselves deficient in some way and go to great extents to hide their flaws. People needing this medicine often have acne or warts and love or hate garlic and onions.

Kelsey's two-month follow-up visit was quite encouraging. "I'm not feeling as depressed. My disposition is a lot better. I'm not so self-conscious and everything seems easier." Her mind was no longer cloudy. She had begun jogging daily. Overall she felt much more positive about herself and less worried about details. "I'm able to focus more and can get a lot more done. I don't care as much about others taking me the wrong way."

At her appointments three and seven months later, Kelsey continued to feel very good. She no longer wore baggy clothing and the feelings of unworthiness were gone. Her only complaint was not having time for a boyfriend. She has not needed another dose of the *Thuja*, has not felt a need for further appointments and is making plans to become a homeopathic physician.

17 The Challenges of Growing Up

Melancholy and Despair in Children and Adolescents

The Carefree Years

Kids are supposed to be happy and full of fun, light-hearted, high-spirited and carefree. Unfortunately, this is not true in all cases. Although an average of 1% of children and 4% of adolescents suffer from depression, depressed adolescents have a 15 to 20% likelihood of suffering from major depression at some point during their adult lives. (Birmaher, et al., p. 1427) Kids tend to experience more separation anxiety, phobias, physical symptoms and behavioral problems, while depression, psychosis and suicide attempts increase with age. (Birmaher, et al., p. 1428) Many children suffering from depression have other problems such as anxiety, substance abuse and conduct problems. A surprisingly high percentage of depressed teenagers, ranging from 20 to 40%, go on to develop bipolar disorder.

A recent study revealed that adolescent girls are far more likely to suffer from depression than their male counterparts. The study, presented to a meeting of the American Psychological Association, attributed the sharply higher rate of depression in girls to *rumination*, which was defined as "passive repetitive focus on negative emotions". Prior to the age of eleven, girls and boys apparently have fairly equal rates of depression, after which point the girls are much more affected by the doldrums. While both sexes reported about the same degree of concern about school, relationships with parents and future career plans, the girls reported many other worries that never even fazed the boys. These included appearance, personal problems, friends, romantic relationships, popularity and safety. The only topic that concerned the boys more than the girls was sports. ("Girls Are Depressed Because They Worry Too Much," *Seattle Times*, p. A3)

An individual episode of depression generally lasts from seven to nine months in children and teenagers and about two-thirds of young people with major depression recover within a year.

(Birmaher, et al., p. 1429) But even after the child feels happier, interpersonal difficulties often persist and the chance of a recurrence of depression is up to 80% within the next five years. (Kah and Michael, p. 60) We feel an urgency about treating depressed kids and teenagers. The longer they feel unhappy, the more their self-image will be affected and the more ingrained depression can become in their psyches. The more quickly we can help them feel better with homeopathy, the greater their chances of lifelong happiness and well-being.

Some kids become depressed with good reason, such as abuse, neglect, poverty, obesity, ridicule or physical illness. It is no surprise that depression tends to run in families. Overall, children of depressed parents are three times more likely to experience a major depression sometime during their lives. The risk is even greater when both parents have mood disorders (Birmaher, et al., p. 1431) The reverse is also true. Depressed kids have a 20 to 46% chance of having depressed parents or siblings. Life situations or events such as alcoholism, drug abuse, sexual or physical abuse, death of a close friend or family member, conflict, difficulty in school or with communication and a poor self-image can all unleash an underlying tendency to suffer from depression.

Children are often less likely than adults to talk about their feelings, particularly if they perceive them to be negative or undesirable. This is especially true in children who may hide their emotions or appear macho, or who have been discouraged from expressing their feelings openly. Any child who appears consistently sullen or withdrawn, who talks about being unwanted, wanting to be dead, or wishing he was never born, or who refers to himself as stupid, good for nothing or having no friends, is probably depressed. These youngsters should be encouraged to openly express their feelings, concerns and dreams, both to parents and, if appropriate, to a psychotherapist, school psychologist or psychiatrist specializing in children.

Any suggestions or threats of suicide should be taken very seriously. The suicide rate among adolescents in this country quadrupled from 1950 to 1996 and suicide is responsible for 12% of teenage deaths. (Birmaher, et al., p. 1430) Certain cultures, such as Japan's, make adolescents even more susceptible to suicide. In 1995, for example, at least ten Japanese school-aged boys took their own lives as a result of being teased, tormented or ostracized by other children. (Reichenberg-Ullman and Ullman, p. 246) The vulnerability and impressionability of children and adolescents can make them highly susceptible to copycat suicides.

Adolescence is a time when youngsters tend to become more independent, communicate more with friends and less with parents, become sexually interested, be exposed to drugs and alcohol for the first time and begin to face the emotional, academic and interpersonal challenges of life. Many parents complain of feeling more distant and alienated from their teenagers. All of these reasons make it even more important for parents to try to maintain a close relationship with their adolescent children and to foster open communication regardless of whether what they have to say is what you want to hear. Some of our patients tell their kids, "You'll never get in trouble with us as long as you tell the truth." This is prudent advice.

No antidepressant has ever been formally approved for children or adolescents even though Prozac and others are prescribed for children with some frequency. Eli Lilly, the manufacturer of Prozac, has submitted data to the Food and Drug Administration (FDA) in an effort to seek approval for the pediatric usage of the drug. Similarly, Smithkline Beecham is analyzing results of its studies on using Paxil with adolescents, Bristol-Myers Squibb with Serzone, and American Home Products with Effexor. (Strauch, p. Al, A19)

FDA approval, however, is not necessary, as evidenced by the nearly 600,000 children and adolescents who received prescriptions for Prozac, Paxil and Zoloft in 1996. In fact, Prozac prescriptions for thirteen- to eighteen-year-olds increased 46% in the same year, boosting total sales figures in the United States to

$1.73 billion. (Strauch, p. Al, A19) Despite these stunning figures, the adult market for Prozac actually declined 5% in 1996 and 2.7% in 1994, leading Eli Lilly to seek out new customers. Some manufacturers of antidepressants are already preparing them in mint- and orange-flavored liquid versions. (Strauch, p. Al, A19) A colleague of ours recently heard that antidepressant bubble gum is also on the drawing board.

Widespread prescribing of antidepressants to children will undoubtedly draw mixed reviews from parents, children, physicians, mental health professionals and educators, much like the response to Ritalin (methylphenidate) for attention deficit hyperactivity disorder (ADHD).

"I Never Let Myself Cry in Front of Anyone"

We first saw Cyndi when she was a fifteen-year-old freshman at a Texas high school. Now, five years later, she has matured into a lovely, talented young woman with an excellent head on her shoulders. Back then she told us, "Everybody thinks I'm a little weird. I dress differently, do things differently. My family calls me "the hippie". I like '60s clothes and big jewelry. I wear black a lot. I'm kind of an artist. I like to read a lot, especially science fiction and romance novels. I have a 4.0 grade-point average. Even in my school I'm considered the odd person. I'm not a preppie or a farm girl.

"I've had a couple of anxiety attacks lately — a feeling in my gut that something is really wrong. My heart starts to beat really fast. It happens when I try to go against my basic beliefs. Like when one of my friends wants me to do something that I know is wrong. Once I kept a friend's secret that she was sleeping with her boyfriend. When her parents found out, I felt guilty and numb.

"I'm a very sensitive person. My friends come to me for advice. Criticism affects me more than it should. How can I fix this? I'm the youngest of three. My childhood was pretty happy. My grandpa died a couple of years ago; then a guy in our class died. I don't usually cry like this in front of other people. I try hard to never let myself cry in front of anyone. I don't know why.

126

Depression comes really easily to me. I'm down all of a sudden. It can turn around really fast. I become very introspective and start wondering what I'm going to do with my life. Music affects me a lot. If I listen to "up" music, it makes me feel good. If I'm depressed, I listen to music to fit my mood and I feel worse."

Cyndi had a tendency to be claustrophobic and feared needles and blood. Once she fainted in a hospital upon seeing an amputee. Ever since their house was robbed, she made sure to lock all the doors whenever she was home alone. Cyndi complained of an occasional rash and of facial acne. She loved pasta and was "grossed out by the fat on meat".

We have given Cyndi ten doses of the same medicine, *Natrum muriaticum*, over the past five years. Each time she has benefited significantly. This is a commonly prescribed medicine for sensitive, introspective people who are particularly sensitive to hurt, criticism, rejection and disappointment. They share the tendencies of not wanting to cry in front of others, of becoming confidantes for their friends, of playing morose music when they feel sad and of loving pasta and hating fatty meat.

The *Natrum muriaticum* has consistently helped to lift Cyndi's moods, brighten her spirits, soothe her disappointments and calm her anxiety and fears. She has weathered many emotional ups and downs, including the death of a close family member, quite well. Her acne has responded to homeopathy, as have various minor complaints over the years. She has become much more emotionally stable and independent. Cyndi has just completed interior design school and is engaged to be married. She has her moments of sadness due to the fact that her fiancé is in the military in the Middle East for two years, but overall she is quite content with herself and her life.

"I Miss My Real Mommy"

Brianna, a sweet five-year-old, was brought in by her adoptive mom, with whom she and her sister had lived since Brianna was three. Her mother shared with us Brianna's story.

127

"She was afraid of all kinds of things when she first came to live with me. At first she had nightmares about losing her birth mom and losing me. She could see a dog two blocks away and she'd leap into my arms. Brianna's the more emotionally fragile of the two. Things make her feel sad instead of mad. She's very quick to cry. Brianna has needed lots of reassurance to try new things and to trust people. Even standing up to her sister has been a major problem."

The product of a blended family, Brianna had a rough start. Both parents were drug and alcohol abusers. She witnessed her birth mother try to slit her wrists. Brianna shared with us: "It was scary. The cops took her. I'm afraid she'll die someday. Sometimes I dream that I'm with her, then a giant spider comes and kills her. I still think about her a lot. I came out of her uterus. I'm just adopted, you know. It's scary because I can't be with my real mommy. I just love her the best."

Brianna's adoptive mom told us that Brianna cried over the smallest things. "I'd describe her as tender-hearted, thoughtful and reflective. She goes through deep periods of grief about her mother. Sometimes she cries so hard that she shakes. She'll be okay for a while, then her sadness gets triggered again. Her memory is so vivid. Brianna can recall every moment of her mother's suicide attempt. When she first came to live with me, she regressed and I had to give her a bottle at night. It took about ten months until she felt bonded to me. I get the impression that she thinks about her mother all the time. She even prays for her at night."

The main physical problem for Brianna was chronic ear infections. Not only was she tenderhearted, but tender headed. She could barely stand for her mom to brush her hair.

A well-known homeopathic medicine for sensitive, sweet, moody, weepy little girls is *Pulsatilla* (wind flower). Each time we have given Brianna this medicine she has become happier, less overly sensitive and less weepy. She has stood up for herself more with her sister and with other children. She no longer falls apart over little things, thinks much less frequently about her birth mother, and when she does think about her, Brianna feels less sad about the situation. Brianna has bonded quite well with her adoptive mom. She no longer pines over her birth mother. Anytime she has experienced ear pain, it has rapidly resolved with a dose of *Pulsatilla*.

"His Grandfather Died at the Very Moment That He Was Conceived"

We had treated Jeremy's mom, a policewoman from Vancouver, successfully for her asthma, so she brought in her sixteen-year-old son, who was also asthmatic. "For a young person," she explained, "he has some very unusual fears. On the freeway driving to the appointment, he kept worrying that there would be an earthquake. Whenever he goes into a room, he immediately begins to think of ways he can get out in case of a tremor. Jeremy worries that he'll be homeless when he grows up. A natural athlete, he's not suited for team sports. He's both sensitive and inconsiderate. And he loves steak.

"My father died of cancer at the exact moment that Jeremy was conceived. I went through a lot of grief. Then, when I was three months pregnant with him, we moved to Nevada and I became terribly homesick. My asthma became worse, and I was on Prednisone during the last half of the pregnancy.

"It was hard to feel like a successful mom with Jeremy. Squawky and dissatisfied, he decided he was finished nursing at nine months. His father and I divorced. Jeremy sees him once or twice a month. His teachers consider him to be borderline attention-deficit disorder because he never works up to his potential and is easily distracted. He's a gifted child with a learning disability. His IQ is over 130. His grade-point average on his last report card was 2.87. Jeremy worries about not knowing what he wants to be when he grows up.

"My child was sexually abused for a period of time by a teenage girl when he was five years old and living with his father and his father's girlfriend. After that his behavior deteriorated. He became furious, aggressive and started hitting other children at school. He was afraid that if he told me I wouldn't let him see his father again, but he did finally confide in me.

"Life looks bleak to Jeremy. You could create a special day just for him, and if one little thing went wrong that's all he would talk about. For Jeremy, there's never enough love to go around. What a moody kid! On the other hand, he's very musical and creative. He makes up his own melodies and he writes poems, too. We've been really close. Jeremy suffered a lot a few years ago when his grandmother died. All in all, he's really a terrific kid."

Jeremy suffered from allergies, chronic sinus problems and asthma. He had scoliosis ever since a bad fall at the age of ten. Asked if he was any different following the injury, his mother acknowledged that he became more withdrawn and reticent. "He was even thinking of killing himself a couple of years ago. He jumped out of the second story of our house but fortunately was not hurt."

"Jeremy's father was a real airhead. He did lots of drugs before we conceived [Jeremy]. His father and stepfather both knocked him around. Jeremy's stepfather felt rejected by him, so he turned around and rejected Jeremy. It's a no-win situation for both of them."

Paintball shooting was Jeremy's absolute favorite thing to do. Although his biggest fear was getting badly hurt or crippled, Jeremy also enjoyed doing dangerous things like cliff climbing and riding his bike downhill without the brakes. He liked shooting and often dreamed of guns. What worried Jeremy the most was losing his friends.

There is an excellent homeopathic medicine for people who are both very sensitive and push the envelope of safety, who feel scorned by those they love and who have a history of head injury and a tendency to suffer from asthma. It is *Natrum sulphuricum* (sodium sulfate), and that is what we prescribed for Jeremy.

Six weeks later Jeremy's sinuses were much improved. He felt happier and could think more clearly. His mother found him to be more reasonable and less of a daredevil. "He's not looking on the dark side. Jeremy's doing really well at his job. He seems to have more energy, even after working a long day. He's much less depressed and he's even more willing to help around the house." Both mother and son were pleased with the results.

Two months later Jeremy continued to do well. He had a partial relapse seven months later due to serious problems between his mother and stepfather, at which time we repeated the medicine. We last saw Jeremy three months ago. He was coping remarkably well with his parents' separation. He told us that he was too busy to be depressed. His mother commented that he was doing well with his friends and making good choices for himself. Now, eighteen months after we first treated him, Jeremy's only problem is mild teenage acne. He has adjusted quite well to his parents' divorce and is a wonderful support for his mother.

PART IV

Homeopathic Treatment of Other Mental and Emotional Problems

18 Nervous, Sleepless and Full of Worry

Anxiety As a Way of Life

How would it feel to worry incessantly, rarely experience a sense of inner peace, feel a constant underlying insecurity, and have an inability to trust that everything will work out for the best without your controlling and micromanaging every last detail. If you suffer from anxiety, this is what your world is like.

If your anxiety is mild, the nervousness and restlessness would be limited to certain situations and exacerbated by only one or a few circumstances. If your anxiety is extreme, you may find yourself in a perpetual state of discomfort, jitteriness and edginess. You may worry to excess about the tiny details of life, which would not even occur to a relaxed person. Living in the present may appear to be impossible due to obsessing about an imagined, unsafe and uncertain future. The over concern may extend beyond the waking hours to sleep, resulting in insomnia, tossing and turning and mulling over worries and insecurities all night. Whether the specific worry is safety for yourself, your family or the world, finances and job security, relationships, health or the anticipation of a particular event, calmness and acceptance seem unattainable. Apprehension, worry, and a sense of foreboding or doom may lurk around every corner. As quickly as one fear or worry is resolved, another erupts.

One of the challenges of conventional treatment of anxiety is the difficulty of separating the effects of anxiety-allaying drugs from a placebo response. Just talking to a doctor or therapist about one's problems may have a very calming effect, perhaps as much so as popping a pill. In fact, in the past fifteen years, researchers in the United States have spent hundreds of millions of dollars on the development of anti-anxiety medications and only one medicine, BuSpar, has won FDA approval. (Schweizer and Rickels, p. 30) Many potential anti-anxiety drugs do no better than placebo in clinical trials.

Though it would be very naive to suggest that homeopathic physicians do not face the same problem in separating out the placebo response with anxious patients, there are measures we use for determining whether our homeopathic medicines are effective. Since homeopathy treats the individual's physical as well as mental and emotional complaints, we expect physical improvement in addition to a lessening of anxiety. If you, as a patient, return after homeopathic treatment saying your anxiety is much less, we ask also about your headaches, joint pain and any other physical problems. We inquire about your general condition such as tolerance to temperature, energy level, quality of sleep, appetite, thirst and cravings for particular foods and drinks. If you report to us that many of your particular problems with these are also significantly lessened, we know it is probable that the homeopathic medicine has alleviated the anxiety rather than crediting only the mere comfort and satisfaction provided by our listening to your story and prescribing treatment. We know that physical symptoms may improve via the placebo response, but if physical changes are not particularly expected by a patient whose chief complaint is anxiety, the improvement is less likely to be the result of placebo alone.

"I Never Felt Safe"

Jackie, a patient of ours for eight years, first sought help at age twenty-two for fatigue, depression and recurrent vaginal infections. A dance teacher, she found her life tiring. All she wanted to do was lie down. Having been previously diagnosed with a systemic yeast infection, she was also annoyed by frequent gas and bloating. In addition, she suffered from painful uterine cramps during her menstrual periods.

Everything in Jackie's life felt like a struggle. Unmotivated and lacking in vitality, she experienced an overall hopelessness about things ever getting better. She feared that the depression would never lift and she would be unable to take care of herself. An overall feeling of discontentment and impatience was present.

After her parents divorced, when Jackie was two years old, the family had moved a lot. The youngest of three, Jackie was known as the serious child of the family. Her mother, an alcoholic, was never available emotionally. A deep, withdrawn child, Jackie was very vulnerable to hurt feelings and grew up feeling uncomfortable with intimacy and affection. Two years after beginning homeopathic treatment Jackie developed a severe psoriasis of the scalp and abdomen. She was disturbed by the dryness, itching, flakiness and tight feeling of her scalp. The patches of eruptions on her abdomen were red, blotchy, scaly and dry.

Although the psoriasis and dark moods were lessened with *Graphites* (graphite), the medicine needed to be repeated more often than usual, leading us to think that a different medicine might produce a more lasting result. It was at this time that Jackie's psoriatic scales became more leathery and the areas burned. When we delved more deeply into Jackie's fears, she confided in us an underlying insecurity stemming from childhood. When she was six years old, a man in a park had exposed himself to her. Embarrassed to share it with her family, her primary feeling was one of being un-protected. Jackie feared that someone would break into her house. She did not feel safe. This generalized insecurity caused her to worry in adulthood about finances, the future and about change in general.

As we explored further, Jackie explained that growing up was very chaotic. With the divorce and all of the moves, nothing felt consistent or predictable. The world was a frightening place to be. She realized that it was no accident that she and her family now were living on an island off the coast of Canada. "I feel pretty safe on the island. When I leave I become afraid of aggressors and attackers. I guess I don't trust people very easily. When I go off-island, I have lots of thoughts and daydreams about someone hurting me or my son. When I visit my relatives, the distrust really comes out. The whole issue growing up was that my family wasn't around much. Mother was busy and I felt abandoned. My stepfather was physically abusive toward my mother. The violence scared me terribly. I just remember being a frightened, depressed little kid. I never felt anyone was there to protect me. It still brings up a lot of grief to think about it. I lived in a constant state of fear."

Jackie's deep-seated fears and depression had their root in her early childhood feelings of abandonment and lack of protection. She has been helped tremendously over the years by *Arsenicum album* (arsenic). This is one of the most commonly used homeopathic medicines for anxiety, insomnia, nervousness, restlessness and a profound underlying fear of dying or being out of control. Not only have Jackie's psoriasis and other physical complaints been relieved by 80 to 90% but the overall feelings of anxiety and hopelessness have been as well. She has generally needed a repetition of the medicine two to three times a year and each time has responded extremely well. We have also been able to give her two children an excellent start in life by treating them homeopathically from the very beginning.

"Mommy, What If You Die While I'm at School?"

Trevor was an unusually nervous kindergartner. With good reason, since there were eight deaths in his family during the six months before he started school. The day before his first day of kindergarten, Trevor was invited to a birthday party. He cried and cried because he didn't want to go. On his big number-one day at kindergarten, the teacher chastised Trevor for arriving two minutes late. Then he felt intimidated by the big kids. By the time his mother left, he was a full-blown basket case. Consumed by pitiful weeping and wailing, poor Trevor felt worse and worse every day. He sobbed with dry heaves. Trevor's teacher, unable to comprehend his reluctance to pass through the schoolroom door, sent him to the principal's office, which of course terrified the child even more. At this point little Trevor refused to speak all day, quite a feat for a kindergartner.

Fortunately, two weeks later Trevor's mom was able to find a different school with a more compassionate teacher. After a few minutes of crying, Trevor decided that he liked the new school better. The year actually progressed well for Trevor and he was overjoyed to be home with his mom over the summer.

First grade was another story. Very nervous again the first day of school, he complained of pain in his stomach when having a bowel movement. As the days progressed, Trevor's anxiety grew worse and he began to fall apart over little things. In kindergarten he had worried that there were fifteen kids in his class; now there were double that number in his first-grade classroom.

Trevor's fears became more generalized. Now he was terrified of meeting new people, of forgetting something he needed to take to school and of getting into trouble. Even though he loved to draw, he worried that he wouldn't do it perfectly and people would yell at him and wouldn't love him.

One day another parent accused Trevor of hitting and spitting on her child, and threatened to sue his family if those behaviors persisted. Although his report cards were flawless, Trevor was devastated when the teacher sent a note home to his parents one time for bad behavior. When the school lost his class picture, he was convinced that he must have done something wrong. He blamed himself when he inadvertently left his show-and-tell folder at home. Nail biting came next. Once, the poor child felt so confused and anxious at school that he kicked his teacher. Trevor developed an increasing tendency to have stomach aches and occasional stomach flus.

By the time Trevor's mom found us, matters were even worse. On the way to school, he complained, "I'm going to have a heart attack! What if you die while I'm at school or somebody breaks in the house?" Trevor insisted that his mom and only his mom drive him to school. His father, who also had a history of school phobia, had less patience with Trevor. He yelled at his son for normal boy things, such as climbing on the furniture, and for being too loud in the house. Trevor's sister, as is often the case in such situations, was the model child. "She's the good one, I'm the bad one," he lamented.

We inquired about Trevor's earlier years to try to understand the source of his over-the-top preoccupations. From infancy to age four, he had exhibited an exaggerated need to be held and nursed. Uncomfortable in strange places, he had been extremely clingy and in constant need of consolation, and he wanted to hold his mother's hand at all times. As a toddler

Trevor had once vomited every fifteen minutes for three days. During a recent stomach flu, he vomited twenty times a day! Aware that there is often a correlation between the state of the parent(s) and the state of the child, we inquired about the mother's state of mind during her pregnancy with Trevor. She admitted to feeling very anxious, depressed and worried during the pregnancy. She experienced frequent vomiting, relieved somewhat by ginger tea, during both of her pregnancies.

We gave Trevor *Bismuth subnitricum,* a wonderful homeopathic medicine for anxious children with stomach aches who feel secure only when they are grasping their mothers' hands. Trevor's response was quite immediate. His next day at school went much more smoothly. Less anxious and irritable, he became much more relaxed. Checking his book bag once was all the reassurance he needed. His hypoglycemia, which his mom forgot to mention during his initial appointment, also improved. When we shared with Trevor's mom our reasons for having given him the *Bismuth,* she reported that, during her morning sickness when pregnant with Trevor, she was so distressed that she used to cling to her own mother.

Bismuth has continued to benefit Trevor considerably. During nearly two years of treatment, the medicine has helped relieve both school anxiety and stomach problems. His moods are so much better and his stomach difficulties and hypoglycemia are gone. Trevor is much easier to live with and is having a great time in school. Most importantly, he is worry free, as a child should be. Trevor's brother, who also suffers from school anxiety, has also responded well to *Bismuth,* confirming the hypothesis that particular symptom pictures and their corresponding homeopathic medicines often run in families.

139

19 The Terror of Life

Phobias and Panic Attacks

Perhaps you are one of the many people who would travel by train, bus or foot rather than even consider taking an airplane. You may do nearly anything to avoid bridges, freeways, elevators, crowds or movie theaters — especially if you can't be guaranteed an aisle seat near the back.

Phobias and panic attacks are not logical. If you suffer from them, you will probably be the first to admit that they are illogical and irrational. Nevertheless they can be limiting and even debilitating. Do your children tire of your insisting on driving them the long way to school to avoid that freeway overpass? Is your spouse tearing his hair out because you just can't bear to fly to Paris for your fiftieth wedding anniversary trip that your kids gave you as a surprise?

A panic attack, which is the main feature of panic disorder, is characterized by a specific episode of intense fear or discomfort in which cardiac (heart palpitations, chest pain or discomfort, sweating and chills or hot flushes), neurologic (dizziness, fainting, numbness, trembling or shaking), gastrointestinal (nausea or abdominal discomfort), and/or respiratory (shortness of breath and a sensation of suffocating or choking) symptoms develop quite suddenly and reach a peak within ten minutes. (Hirschfeld, p. 3) They are accompanied by a strong fear of losing control or dying.

Recent figures indicate that more than one in every six people will have at least one sudden experience of unexplained fear in their lifetime. More than 11% of the population will suffer four or more of the physical symptoms mentioned and about half of those who have such a fearful spell may later have panic attacks, often recurrent. Women are two and a half times more likely to develop panic attacks than men. The most common time of onset is between the ages of twenty-five and thirty-four for women and thirty and forty-four for men. (Hirschfeld, p. 4–5) Panic disorder is often hereditary and its onset often occurs during times of stress or hormonal fluctuation. Recent evidence suggests that only half of people with panic disorder seek help and that panic disorder may be linked to childhood sexual abuse. (Katerndahl, p. 275)

Judyth learned about panic attacks firsthand. "I am a seasoned traveler, having flown long distances, often across continents, for decades without a second thought. Then, four years ago, I sat aboard a plane on my way to a meeting in the Midwest. We had just bought a new home and I really wanted to stay with Bob to plan the decor. A colleague headed for the same meeting was sitting farther back in the plane. The air was hot and stuffy, and my seat was situated in the middle of the plane, by a window seat next to a very large woman.

"All of a sudden I became unexplainably nervous and claustrophobic. I simply felt that I must get out of the plane. The doors to the aircraft were closed, but we weren't yet moving. I sheepishly explained to the attendant that I had flown many times before without any problem but that I was feeling nervous and didn't think I could handle flying. She reassured me that I would be fine and suggested that I try to relax. Gripped with fear, relaxing seemed absolutely out of the question. I took a few deep breaths, which had been my usual way to sink into a state of calmness. It didn't work and I felt worse by the minute, or maybe even by the second. The plane edged its way down the runway and we were next in line for takeoff.

"I scarcely remember what happened next, probably because it was so embarrassing. I got up and told the attendant that I just didn't think I could continue the flight. To this day no one believes my story, but somehow the plane turned back and dropped me off at the gate. I vaguely remember asking the attendant to let my colleague know what happened. I have no idea how I even got my checked luggage. Back in the airport I called Bob and still remember his shock. 'You did WHAT? You MUST be kidding!' Unfortunately, thanks to me, the plane arrived twenty minutes late and no one ever notified my puzzled colleague why I was no longer on the plane!

"I have flown many times on both short and very long flights since then and have never avoided any flights based on that experience. A physician friend prescribed a mild tranquilizer for flight anxiety, which I have never taken. Most of the time I'm fine, though I do occasionally have moments of mild anxiety. On occasion I have taken a homeopathic *Aconitum napellus* (monkshood), which has quickly allayed my discomfort. Fortunately, I have never again had to make a plane turn back! Nor have I been tempted to disembark, even during 22-hour flights to India, with lots of intermediate stops. I wondered for a moment when Bob and I flew standby on a flight from the Bay Area to Seattle and were assigned the two seats at the very rear of the plane. But I was still fine.

"My panic attack gave me tremendous insight into what my patients and others experience. Now I understand that unreasonable fears and phobias can happen to anyone, even me. And at those times when I have had the courage to share my story with others, I have been amazed at how many people, even frequent fliers, have had similar experiences."

"Get Me Out of Here: Anyplace but an Airplane"

Sally, a thirty-four-year-old public relations consultant, sought out homeopathy for relief from her panic attacks. British and very accustomed to transcontinental air travel, she had become more and more nervous over the past few years about flying. Her anxiety had increased considerably following a stillbirth a year earlier. The night before the delivery, after she and her husband learned their baby had died, she shook all night. These shaking fits recurred several times after that but were now associated in her mind with flying to Europe. The panic attacks were characterized by extreme anxiety and violent heart palpitations from which Sally felt as if her heart would jump right out of her chest.

Prior to her daughter's death, Sally experienced occasional panicky thoughts, such as wondering what would happen if her car plunged off a bridge, but she could dismiss them. Now she felt forced to work through the entire scenario, such as a flight, in order to cope. If the thought of her car falling off the bridge entered her mind, she felt compelled to imagine the car sinking into the water, being unable to open the doors, trying to figure out how to open the windows and having only seconds to save her own or her husband's life. Sally's feeling was sheer terror. What if she couldn't escape? What if she made the wrong decision and one or both of them died as a result?

Sally's greatest fear about flying was the anticipation of the crash — knowing that something was wrong and waiting for it to happen. She became extremely edgy if the plane experienced any turbulence or if a bell was supposed to go off but didn't. The only way she could become calm was to remind herself that she had absolutely no control over the situation.

Her fears had begun to multiply. Riding in the passenger seat of a car, Sally replayed the bridge scenario. If she had to stay in a hotel she worried about a disastrous fire. Concerns about her health had also become magnified. What if she suffered a heart attack? Or breast cancer? No one could tell her why her daughter died. Maybe she, too, had something terribly wrong with her and no one knew. Since the stillbirth, Sally had lost confidence in doctors.

Sally was plagued by a deep sense of failure since the baby's death. Having a child was what she had planned for her life and it didn't happen even though she thought she had done everything right. She lived in fear of others asking her if she had any children. "I'm wondering if the grass is greener. I have a good marriage, I enjoy my life and my job, but I'm great at living for tomorrow. When we travel, I drive my husband crazy. He makes the arrangements with the travel agent, then I go over the whole list, one by one, to make sure he's made the best connections. I like to check it all out."

Fortunate enough to have had a happy childhood on a farm in the English Lake District, Sally had a very stable upbringing. But despite her carefree beginnings, Sally was forever worrying about one thing or another. If it was not fear that something terrible would happen to her husband, it was concern that she might die in a future childbirth, as did a family friend. "My imagination just goes wild. I tend to take little things and blow them way out of proportion." Sometimes Sally's anxiety caused her to wake every hour on the hour. She frequently awoke in the middle of the night, thought she heard a strange sound, then convinced herself that a robber was breaking in and would kill the family. Then she quickly imagined herself racing to the phone, dialing 911, and running to the door. She admitted to a having a dreadful fear of her own mortality. Physical problems included periodic rashes and herpes on the face. Also troubling were her menstrual periods, which had become considerably heavy and clotted and lasted longer. She was bothered also by a persistent vaginal discharge. She loved coffee, chocolate and bread.

Sally matched the picture of *Argentum nitricum* (silver nitrate). This is a medicine for people with anticipatory anxiety of all kinds. They often have claustrophobia and a fear of heights and bridges. Those needing this medicine have a perpetual tendency to imagine disasters and catastrophes and, therefore, are likely candidates for phobias and panic attacks. Sally's five-week follow-up report was very positive. She felt much less anxious about flying and had flown from Seattle to Chicago without incident. The thoughts about driving off a bridge were gone as were the palpitations. The insomnia was somewhat alleviated. Sally had a small patch of ringworm for the first time in twenty years. Since she had it all the time as a child, we understood that this symptom was part of her healing response and that it would resolve over time.

Over the past three years Sally has continued to do extremely well. She has needed six doses of the *Argentum nitricum* and continues to feel very good. She has two lovely children, one of whom we have treated successfully with homeopathy for recurrent ear infections.

"Do I Need to Go to a Mental Hospital?"

We first met Irene, "just sixty-three", seven years ago. A German woman "from the old country", we liked her the moment we met her. Vibrant and friendly, she had been treated by various holistic physicians for nearly fifteen years. Irene complained of fatigue, weakness of the lower limbs, depression, allergies, tension headaches, gas and recurrent colds even though she was "healthy as a horse".

Irene described herself as "high-strung, intense and emotional. I get too emotional and tend to baby people. I used to hate yearly good-byes after I visited my mother in Germany. I'm an idealist. I feel things deeply. I never feel like I do enough. I seem to worry about everything — about my family, getting skin cancer, hospitals, death. When I feel afraid, I get a nervous stomach and I stutter. Lately I've felt a sitting-on-the-edge-of-my-chair impatience, like nothing's going fast enough. And lately I feel confused and absentminded, as if I were in a fog.

"The past two months have been especially stressful for me. I've been feeling panicky, helpless, not in control of my health or my body. I wake at three in the morning with a dry mouth and a racing heart, worrying if I'm going to get sick and who's going to help me. Who will manage my life? What doctor should I see? Who should I call? Do I need to go to a mental hospital? Is it a heart attack? A stroke?" This was the first time Irene had ever known panic attacks. Before she had just plain worried.

"I'm afraid to go to work or to be alone. It's an anxiety unlike any I've ever had before. I've started to get hot, needlelike sensations when I feel this way or after dinner. I feel jittery. My brain is just going. My stools are loose and I have a nervous stomach and nervous chills. I feel touchy, irritable, and I can't stand noise. I feel so hungry. Am I going to have a nervous breakdown? Am I going nuts?"

This is a classic panic attack for which the most appropriate medicine is *Arsenicum album*, which we mentioned in the preceding chapter. It fit Irene's exact symptoms perfectly. She called four days after taking a single dose of the medicine to report that her heartbeat was less rapid and the anxiety attacks much improved. At her visit six weeks later, she reiterated that the medicine "worked fine. I've gotten rid of the early-morning attacks. I've felt really relaxed. This is how I'm supposed to be. My bowel movements are a lot more regular. I'm not jittery. The chills are gone, my appetite is good and I'm no longer afraid of being alone. I'd say I feel 70% better. I've never felt this calm."

We repeated the medicine four and a half months later because Irene felt the effects were waning. She still felt much better than when we first saw her. She did not experience fearfulness, weakness in the legs, headaches or worries about her health, but the jitteriness returned a bit, her pulse was up and down, and she had awakened once again at 3 A.M. Her calmness returned after the second dose.

We didn't see Irene again for five years because she felt fine. She had returned then in a panic similar to the first time we saw her. She was preoccupied as before about getting sick with no one to take care of her. Irene's husband had suffered from shingles. The medication he was given precipitated hallucinations. Understandably, Irene plunged into her first panic attack in five years. We gave her another dose of the *Arsenicum album* and saw her five weeks later. "No palpitations, no headaches, energy way up, no worrying about anything. I'm not picking up on others' nervousness and I'm able to cope just fine. I'd say I'm 100% better." That was eight months ago and Irene has not needed any further treatment. Hopefully this last dose of the *Arsenicum* will last another five years or more!

A Rich Fantasy Life

Cat, a thirty-year-old dentist from Boston, came to us for help with asthma and panic attacks. "I'm sensitive to a number of different foods, especially dairy products. I think I'd call it a sensitivity or irritability to the world in general. I have dark circles under my eyes, even when I follow my rigid diet. My asthma gets worse when I think about it, like when I lie in bed at night. Then I start to panic and shake. I had a really bad experience with an inflamed knee. The orthopedic physician gave me a cortisone injection and I had a terrible reaction. Now I have to walk with special orthotics. I'm scared to hike. I can feel a sensation in my knee.

"It scares me. First the asthma, then the knee and then panic attacks. Now my left shoulder is starting to fitz out on me. How far will it go? Will I be dead by the time I'm forty? I'm better adjusted than almost anyone I know. How can all of these things happen to me? Am I somehow inviting them into my life?"

We asked Cat to tell us when the panic attacks began. "Five years ago I was engaged to be married. Three weeks before the wedding I felt terribly trapped and canceled the whole thing. It was at that time that I flew to Texas to be with my family and felt a sudden tingling all over my body. I was so claustrophobic by the time I got to the Dallas airport that I ran out." Cat also described a fear of drowning in deep water.

"Since that time, I have these periods where I'm almost manic. Especially since I've become fascinated with short stories and books about fantasy. I get to feeling quite elevated and full of creative ideas and I don't feel like going to sleep. I feel sometimes like the mania is right behind me; like I could enter into a manic state just like someone brushes her teeth. All of my problems are mental and emotional like most well-adjusted people. I'm vital, out there, easily excitable. I can be a marshmallow on the inside but people see my fiery nature.

"When I was twelve my family moved from Vermont to Texas. Life in Vermont was idyllic. The move totally destroyed me. A few months later my mind split and I went into a fantasy world. I started having daydreams about characters in novels. Now, decades later, my daydreams are entire stories with well developed characters and plots. The more I developed as a person, the more the characters did, too. I started reading more and more fiction. In fact, I'm hoping to write a fantasy book myself.

"I get such vivid pictures in my head. I can taste the apple, feel the chair. The daydreams are so incredible that I feel like I'll explode. But it's all pictures. I can't understand how people have words in their heads. I'll be driving to the office and a tomato flashes in my mind, and I start thinking of all the implications of 'tomato'. I began drinking massive amounts of caffeinated drinks all day long. Some days I'll drink about thirty-two ounces of iced tea. I think I've totally destroyed my liver with all of the caffeine. I prefer tea to coffee because coffee gives me bad breath. When I clean house, I reward myself with half an hour of private reverie. When I go to a concert, I can sometimes not even hear a note because I'm lost in my daydreams. My fantasies are incredibly multifaceted. The characters triumph over their problems."

From the time she was a child, Cat had a spirit about her. Independent, happy and witty, she was forever lighthearted and playful. Highly sensitive to noises and other external stimuli, Cat also had a hard time sitting still for very long.

When we inquired about Cat's dreams, she responded, "I don't have too many. I don't want dreams. In fact, I despise them. I want eight hours of complete darkness." Cat must have drawn a fine line, however, between her dreams and her reveries, because as soon as she hit the pillow, she was again deeply enmeshed in elaborate adventures.

A spontaneous woman, Cat built the deep foundation of her life on whims. If it felt right to do something, she would, without thinking. "The reason I thrive talking to people is because that's when I form my thoughts." We looked forward to our conversations with Cat because she was so lively, fascinating and fun — one of our most delightful patients.

In addition to her asthma, Cat had a history of recurrent bladder infections. She loved sweets, salt, alcohol and oily foods.

The more unusual the person, the easier it is to find a homeopathic medicine of great benefit. Cat was definitely a one-of-a-kind person. Her remarkable, vivid fantasies and intense propensity to daydream; her animated, vivacious nature and the predilection for caffeine led us to give her *Coffea* (coffee bean). The discomfort in her chest was alleviated, although at first she was constantly on the alert for "that little wheeze", because she couldn't believe it had gone away. Much calmer, Cat was able to fly with greater peace of mind. She was able to engage in fulfilling intimate relationships. She has needed eight doses of the *Coffea* over the past two and a half years, usually after exposure to aromatic oils. Cat's daydreams continue to be alive and well, and she has continued to put her boundless energy and creativity to good use. She has recently written a fantasy novel of her own.

"I Can't Get Unwound"

Jack, a thirty-eight-year-old investment banker, was very pleasant and immaculately dressed. Married, with four children, he had worked for two prominent banking institutions over the previous sixteen years. "I've simply become way too wound up. My sleep is erratic. I actually went to consult a psychiatrist about a year ago because I felt like my wheels were going off the track. I had a horrible experience with Prozac and other antidepressants. My system is sensitive and I reacted terribly. I guess I found out what I didn't want to do.

"This year has really brought things to a head. I'm very accomplished at what I do. But when I sit down with a prospective investor, my stomach begins to bubble and my heart races. It feels as if I'm losing control of the situation. My whole sense of calm and self-confidence dissolves. I get short with the kids and I'm almost too stressed to enjoy sex. The stress spills out all over my life. I know the wounds are self-inflicted. It's the perception of needing to be successful and compete with people at the upper range of achievement."

Jack was lucky to enjoy very high energy. Up at 5 A.M., he bounced out of bed and was ready to go, without ever needing a caffeine boost. In fact, caffeine "destroyed" Jack. Self-critical by nature, Jack was extremely demanding of himself and his accomplishments. When seized by tension, Jack's breathing became shallow, his back and neck constricted and his stomach felt tight. His psychiatrist likened him to an A student who had to keep up his grades. Losing was a big deal for Jack. As far back as grade school, losing a baseball game was a serious matter. He just got used to winning — in everything. Honest and trustworthy, he had excelled in business. Yet he felt overwhelmed by a fear of being unsuccessful.

Jack's bottom-line feeling was being out of control. No matter how large an account he was able to secure, he continually fixated on "screwing up". Indulging in frequent comparison with his colleagues, his sense of inner calmness evaporated. He was consumed by thought, worry and anticipation. As we interviewed Jack in more depth, we discovered that his first panic attack occurred eighteen years earlier, in his first business class. As he got up in front of a group of thirty or so other students, he became lightheaded, drenched in perspiration, his heart raced and he had to sit down. That incident instilled in him a fear of looking stupid, out of control. What if the situation repeated itself? Over the years it did, so frequently in recent times that he had to find an answer other than antidepressants.

In Jack's case, it took a little over a year to find the medicine that had the most profound effect on him. We first gave him *Nux vomica* (Quaker's button), a homeopathic medicine commonly used for an overstressed, irritable, hard-driving, type-A personality. No success.

We then ascertained that Jack needed one of the medicines made from metals used for individuals who place a very strong emphasis on performance, success and reaching a great height in their career — highly responsible achievers who experience a great fear of falling from the position they have worked so hard to achieve.

Jack's case was a challenge for us. After trying *Titanium, Aurum metallicum, Rhodium* and *Niccolum* (nickel), some of which had a partial effect of helping Jack, we arrived at *Cuprum metallicum* (copper). As with conventional medications, finding the very

150

best homeopathic medicine for an individual can take time, though generally not more than six months.

The main problem for someone needing *Cuprum* is the over-powering desire to maintain control — serious, conscientious, responsible individuals, they push themselves very hard. They make excellent leaders and can be depended upon to follow through with their commitments. These people can have a great fear of heights, which was true of Jack. As a child his most vivid dreams were of falling from a very high place. "I'd wake up before I would go splat." Jack did not suffer from the muscle cramps typical of those needing this medicine, but he did incur an injury to his calf muscle, which had inhibited his running routine.

After taking the *Cuprum*, Jack didn't see us again for five months. A busy, practical fellow, he didn't feel a need to come see us, since he was doing so well. The notion of losing control had rarely even occurred to him. He felt like his old self who didn't get wound up about meetings or presentations. The sensation of observing and judging himself had disappeared. His sleep had also improved. What brought Jack back in to see us was a return of the anxiety — though not as severe as before the *Cuprum* — after he drank coffee at a friend's birthday party a month earlier. He had a meeting with a high-powered client scheduled for the following week and he definitely needed to feel himself again. It was evident to Jack and to us that the coffee had interfered with his progress, so we repeated the medicine, which restored his mental peace. Jack's wife has also benefitted considerably from homeopathic treatment.

20 Living on a Seesaw

The Unpredictability of Mood Swings

The Buddha once said that the only thing that is constant is change. Life is a series of expected and unexpected events. Adjusting, rather than overreacting, to these events is an essential aspect of coping with everyday existence. Being content with life requires a blend of flexibility and stability. The ability to remain calm amid the sometimes stormy waves of life is an invaluable tool.

Mood swings can make you erratic, unstable and even hysterical. The normal happenstances of life may feel like one catastrophe or crisis after another rather than a natural flow of events. It is no fun to be moody. You may wake up in the morning feeling perky, then moments to hours later feel like a crab. Those around you feel as if they are walking on eggshells because they have no idea if you will hug them or jump down their throats. Mood swings are not a good ingredient for making lasting friendships. Your family and friends may try to keep their distance, since they never know what to expect. All around, mood swings are an energy drain that impair your peace of mind. In milder cases of mood swings, referred to in the psychiatric literature as *cyclothymia*, damage to relationships can be caused, as well as to self-esteem and career. These mood changes are not severe enough to be classified as bipolar disorder or major depression but can still interfere considerably with a person's life.

"I Came to You As a Last Resort"

Alicia, a thirty-three-year-old stockbroker, felt "like a zombie" with her migraine headaches, which generally occurred around her periods and had begun when she was twenty. At the time that she first consulted us, in 1991, her head pain was so bad that she literally had to "put one foot in front of the other through sheer will" to function. She took 1,000 milligrams of Tylenol every three to four hours to survive the pain.

"Growing up wasn't very happy for me. During my senior year of high school, I became very depressed after a breakup with my boyfriend. I slept a lot and lost twenty pounds. I did fine during my first year of college and my grade-point average was 3.8." Then, after moving back to Georgia, she started to slide into a deep depression, slept twenty hours a day, rarely bathed or ate, and avoided class. Her grades plummeted to Ds and Fs. She somehow pulled herself through it and graduated from college.

Alicia had two switches: "on" and "off". During her "on" phase, which she described as "hyper", Alicia was fastidious, detail-oriented, assertive, driven and on top of everything. She multi-tasked, talked quickly and her insides churned. Her movements were jerky and speedy. Other people didn't move as fast and make decisions quickly enough. Alicia loved her hyper phase because she accomplished so much. When she was "off", her work stacked up and she couldn't function. Then she felt normal for a week until the cycle would begin again. During her down phase, Alicia "slid down from peak to normal, then hit the wall." She lacked energy, went to bed by seven in the evening and wanted to be left alone. She felt hopeless, helpless and bleak, wondering why she should even keep going.

Compassionate to the extreme, Alicia couldn't bear to listen to the news or hear about abused or neglected children. Seeing a dead animal by the side of the road would propel her into uncontrollable weeping. She wept intensely as she told me about riding in a bus that had killed a dog accidentally. After that incident, Alicia had refused to travel by bus.

Alicia's mother died of metastatic breast cancer at fifty-six, as did her maternal grandmother at thirty-six. Her uncle was diagnosed with prostate cancer at fifty. Alicia feared she, too, would develop cancer. A dermatologist had removed a couple of moles for her, and although they were benign, Alicia had devoured the literature on malignant melanoma. In addition to the migraines, Alicia's problems included dark moles all over her body, chronic strep throat and uterine fibroids resulting in a total hysterectomy a year before we first saw her.

Claustrophobic since she was a little girl, Alicia held her breath and counted while on elevators and got out if there were too many people. She avoided crowded streets and stores and worried excessively about strangers abducting her son.

Alicia's temperature ran hot and cold like her moods. She loved the sun but wilted in extreme heat. She adored Thai noodles, pasta, bread and double lattes.

It was her unbearable migraines that had led Alicia to see us. She hadn't a clue that homeopathy could also help her drastic mood swings. Alicia responded beautifully to *Carcinosin* (a nosode), a medicine for intense, sympathetic individuals with a tendency to have moles and a strong family history of cancer.

At her three-month visit, Alicia reported that she couldn't ever remember feeling so good. The migraines were gone, except for some infrequent, mild aching. Her moods were stable and her stamina was better than ever. Two months later, she still had had no migraines and had experienced only one minor episode of depression.

Alicia continued to feel exceptionally well. Since we first saw her six and a half years ago, she needed only one repetition of the *Carcinosin*. In a letter that she wrote to us several years ago, she described her experience with homeopathy: "I can hardly believe where I was before beginning homeopathy and where I am today. After suffering so many years from the severe mood swings and debilitating migraines, I had nearly given up hope. I came to you as a last resort. I don't honestly think I expected anything near the dramatic results I experienced. I feel really free for the first time. How I lasted as long as I did I'll never know. I tell my story to anyone who indicates the slightest interest!"

"I'm Either Up or I'm Down"

Jimmy, a twenty-six-year-old scriptwriter from Los Angeles sought out homeopathic treatment six years ago for fatigue and a foggy mind. He was taking handfuls of nutritional supplements for digestive discomfort and a recurrent upper-respiratory infection. Rectal itching was another annoyance. In addition, Jimmy showed us a long list of more minor complaints, including headaches, allergies, chemical sensitivities and muscle tightness. All in all, Jimmy felt as if he was "withering away". He had suffered from nosebleeds lasting several days since he was a boy. The episodes, consisting of dark red strings of blood, still occurred unless he took an iron supplement regularly.

Six years earlier Jimmy had lost fifty pounds through dieting but felt weakened in the process. "The last five or six years are a blur. My sense of time and my memory are distorted. I can't tell if I moved to L.A. two weeks or six months ago. My moods alternate. One day I look at a book or listen to music and love it. The next day I hate the same book and music. It's like I'm a different person. I'm like a light switch that's totally on or off. Maybe there's something inside of me that's causing the whole problem. It feels like something is living inside my lower intestines. Sometimes it even feels like it wants to poison me.

"I'm a night person. I prefer to go to sleep when the sun comes up. The night is much quieter and less crowded. My confidence is either too high or too low. I'm either up or down. Either I can't stop joking, laughing and singing, or I'm sad and morose. Can you help me level out?"

One medicine for rapidly alternating, extreme mood swings combined with profuse, often clotted nosebleeds is the plant *Crocus sativa* (saffron). Five weeks after taking a dose of *Crocus* Jimmy felt stronger and more oriented to time and his moods were more stable. His gas was lessened a great deal. Three months passed. Jimmy's mind was more often clear. His moods alternated less. "I feel more focused and much more like myself. My creativity and imagination have returned. My concentration is excellent." Jimmy continued to respond well to the *Crocus* during the year and a half that we treated him.

High on Life

Tom, a forty-seven-year-old commercial architect, was a transplant from Vermont. He and his wife had moved to Seattle three years earlier. "We love this city. It's heavenly! My health is excellent, except for headaches. In fact I feel pretty euphoric about life. With the headaches, I get this light feeling, almost like my feet are floating off the ground.

"I've had some trouble with my mother-in-law. It's been kind of a roller coaster for the past few years. My feelings toward her have been extreme at times — anger, resentment. She belittles me in front of my wife and I don't like it. But I love my job and our home. We have a beautiful view of Puget Sound. It's utopia." We noticed that Tom laughed in a bubbly way as he spoke, a contagious sort of giggle.

"My colleagues call me a visionary. I get wonderful ideas at night during my dreams. It's as if I go to a special place full of creative ideas and bring them all back. My clients love the offices I design. They're airy, with lots of open spaces. You know, if I didn't love my work so much, I think I'd like to be an astronomer. I find myself daydreaming about the universe and black holes and all the bazillions of atoms around us.

"Most of the time I feel really high, but I do have my black moments where I sense a deep loneliness. I worry about getting sick or dying or even going crazy. At those times, like with the headaches, I feel very light, kind of spacey. I can almost feel the space between my cells."

Tom was a fascinating fellow. Highly creative, with brilliant, far-reaching ideas. But he was not grounded. The medicine that benefited him was *Hydrogen*. He remarked at his two-month follow-up appointment: "My headaches are gone. I feel more solid and grounded. The spaces in between my cells have filled in. I don't weigh any more but I feel like I do. This is the old Tom. Consistently happy like I used to be. Not so many ups and downs. I'm no longer afraid of getting sick or going crazy. I feel great."

We gave Tom a second dose of the *Hydrogen* after he received a strong exposure to camphor, which often interferes with homeopathic treatment. It's been a year since we last saw Tom. He has continued to be headache-free, feels much more himself and is still high on life but in a more balanced way.

21 Way Up and Way Down

Overcoming the Roller Coaster of Bipolar Disorder

If depression can be called "being down in the dumps", severe mood swings may be likened to being on an emotional roller coaster. The changeability of temperament, known as lability, can be terribly disturbing, not only to the individual involved but to friends, family and work associates. The degree of unpredictability can be mild or extreme. Family members often describe their feelings about being around the person as "walking on eggshells" or "living with Dr. Jeckyll and Mr. Hyde" because they never know what to expect next.

In bipolar disorder, formerly called manic depression, the effects can be much more devastating even to the point of social isolation, recurrent hospitalizations (the revolving-door syndrome) and even suicide. Symptoms can include an elevated mood lasting over one week, racing thoughts, overabundant energy, diminished need for sleep, rapid and pressured speech, restlessness, hallucinations and/or delusions, grandiosity and low self-esteem. Those with bipolar disorder are known for their excessive activities and habits, including buying sprees, enormous telephone bills, brilliant creative and artistic endeavors, spur-of-the-moment travel or sex, bizarre dress and anything else that catches their fancy.

"Mood disorders are the 'common cold' of major psychiatric illnesses, and more than 20 million Americans will suffer an episode of depression or mania during their lifetimes. One in five families will directly feel their impact." (Papalos and Papalos, p. 3) Bipolar disorders constitute 20% of all major mood disorders. (Appleton, p. 26) Bipolar disorder afflicts equal numbers of women and men and more than a third of all cases surface before age twenty. (Jamison, p. 45) About 15% of people who have experienced a major depression will develop bipolar disorder, equally distributed among men and women. About two thirds of manic episodes occur just before or after a

157

major depression. If left untreated, people with bipolar disorder have approximately four episodes in ten years, the interval decreasing with age. About 80% of these individuals feel normal between episodes. (Appleton, p. 26) Though infrequent, the manic episodes can be enough to sabotage relationships, jobs and happiness.

Bipolar disorder is treated conventionally with lithium carbonate, Depakote, Lamictil, Tegretol, Risperdal, Abilify, Geoden, and Seroquel, as well as antianxiety medications like Klonopin (clonazepam) for the manic phase and an antidepressant for the depressive phase. (Appleton, p. 27) Some 60 to 80% of all adolescents and adults who commit suicide have a history of bipolar disorder or depression. Before the late 1970s, when the drug lithium first became widely available, one person in five with manic depression committed suicide. (Jamison, p. 46)

Bipolar disorder is not a recent phenomenon. Throughout history some very well-known individuals have suffered from this problem: King Saul of the Bible (who needed David's music to soothe his despondency), Abraham Lincoln, Winston Churchill and Theodore Roosevelt. "The writers and poets Johann Goethe, Honoré de Balzac, Leo Tolstoy, Virginia Woolf, Ernest Hemingway, Robert Lowell and Anne Sexton suffered mood swings, as did the composers George Friederich Handel, Robert Schumann, Hugo Wolf, Louis-Hector Berlioz and Gustav Mahler. These people are known and respected, so it may be that the illness fuels a certain kind of drive and creativity. However, a study of their lives would also reveal searing anguish, shattered relationships, psychosis and even suicide." (Papalos and Papolos, p. 4)

The diagnosis of bipolar disorder can be confused with or occur in the same patient as psychosis. This explains why, in the following cases, the patients may have been given antipsychotic medications.

Impulsive, Snappy and Out of Whack

Sandy, a forty-year-old medical receptionist with two young children, had been diagnosed with bipolar disorder and borderline depression. Currently on Zoloft and Paxil, and on Ambien as needed for sleep, lithium had not been of benefit. "I've been diagnosed with lots of things and taken more medications than I can even remember."

"Intense, creative, empathetic, manipulative, strong-willed, judgmental, loyal, stubborn, hot-tempered and impatient" was how Sandy described herself. But most of all, she complained of her impulsivity, which was aggravated by caffeine. "I'm impulsive in my attention, parenting, eating, spending. You name it and I do it impulsively." Her impulsivity had led to scatteredness, frequent job changes and turmoil in her relationships.

Drastic mood fluctuations — from depression to flash temper to impatience — were very disturbing to her. Her black, painful depressions made her feel trapped in a "horrible pit" and led to three suicide attempts, the last having occurred ten years before we first met her. That last attempt was just after the death of her mother, the pillar of her life. Sandy apologized at this point in the interview for jumping from topic to topic while recounting her history. "I've looked forward to this appointment for so long. I wish I could give you a straightforward chronology."

Sandy shared more about her mood swings. "I take on more than I can handle, then I start to lash out. When my anger comes out, I yell at my husband and threaten to divorce him. I think my depression had to do with being rejected. My parents divorced when I was a little girl, and my strict, unloving grandmother came to raise me because my mother had to work full-time. Then a boyfriend ended our relationship when I was fourteen. I went from being a shy, quiet girl to a rebellious teenager. I went from one relationship to another looking for love. That was around the time of my first suicide attempt. I took a bottle of antibiotics on impulse after my mother got really mad at me for staying out too late. Years later my mother married an alcoholic who went from being loving to abusive in minutes. Shortly after, she died of ovarian cancer." Very dependent on her mother, Sandy felt that a part of herself was dying along with her mother. Her mother's death was like a door slamming, leaving her with no one on whom she could lean.

A moment-to-moment person, Sandy acted without thinking and didn't consider goals or long-term consequences. Sticking with anything was extremely challenging. Quite bright, she'd studied physical therapy for a year, then dropped out to get married. Money was also something Sandy couldn't hold onto for long. A spate of bad luck and a habit of buying things before she thought about what she could afford led to financial disaster. "I have a shotgun approach to everything."

Sandy enjoyed mothering but resented the need to mother her husband as well. Her sexual desire was quite low, which distressed both her and her husband. Fearful of falling and of the dark, Sandy suffered from vivid, disturbing dreams about ghosts, of fighting evil forces and of losing her soul. She adored French fries with extra salt, and she could live on bread and butter. Sandy also had a strong desire for stimulants such as caffeine and uppers. Hot weather caused her to suffer from headaches, nausea and diarrhea. Insomnia was a chronic problem, as was nail biting since child-hood. She also complained of a rash under her lips.

Due to her debilitating impulsivity, changeable nature, history of manic and depressive episodes, issues with mothering and her own mother, food cravings and aggravation from the sun, we pre-scribed homeopathic *Lithium muriaticum* (lithium chloride). At her two-month follow-up visit, Sandy was happy to report that her impulsivity had diminished by 90%. She could shop without going crazy, had stopped biting her nails and had lost eight pounds by limiting her carbohydrate consumption. She had decided to eliminate caffeine and was surprised at how energetic she felt.

When Sandy returned three months after her initial appoint-ment, the impulsivity continued to be diminished. She was, however, still quite bothered by premenstrual irritability. "Every little thing bugs me. I pick at my husband. He can't do anything right. I just want him to leave me alone. I even shove away my daughter when she gets too clingy." She also com-plained of fatigue, bloating, nipple tenderness and constipa-tion prior to her periods. Upon questioning Sandy further, she reported significant depression during her two pregnancies. Her sexual energy was nearly nonexistent. She loved to dance and craved chocolate. At this point we gave Sandy a different homeopathic medicine, *Sepia*, predominately for mood shifts due to hormonal shifts. We generally find success with one homeopathic medicine to treat all of an individual's symptoms, however this was a case where two different medicines in succession were quite beneficial.

Two months later Sandy shared that her premenstrual irritability and fatigue were substantially improved. The facial rash was gone and the nipple tenderness was milder and of shorter duration. She noticed that she sometimes started to criticize her husband, then apologized and backed off. Her fuse took longer to light. "I don't rant and rave and rescue anymore." Four months later we gave Sandy a higher dose of the *Sepia* because she still complained about her libido and had even resorted to testosterone injections. She called four weeks later to say that the medicine had worked miraculously. Not only was her depression dramatically reduced but she had retrieved memories of childhood sexual abuse that she felt explained a lot about her history of mood swings.

Now, thirteen months after beginning homeopathic treatment, Sandy continues to feel quite well. She describes the overall improvement as 85 to 90%, depending upon the amount of stress in her life. With homeopathic treatment, her rage is gone, the PMS symptoms dramatically reduced and she feels much happier in her marriage and her life.

"God's Special Child"

Lily, a thirty-five-year-old respiratory therapist from Alabama diagnosed with bipolar disorder some years earlier, has been under our care for the past two years with considerable success. When we first spoke with her, she shared this story: "I'm really struggling. This is the lowest period of my life. My depression has been even worse since I had a miscarriage almost two years ago. I feel so unhappy. I just can't find any joy within myself."

Able to function at work, Lily was caught in the grips of depression the moment she came home. "Dishes in the sink, newspapers on the floor. That's the first thing I see when I walk in the door. Then I have to start cleaning right away. If my kitchen's a mess, my life's a mess. My husband and children can tell you how cranky and unhappy I am around the house. Home is never right. Not the right furniture, nor the right pictures on the walls.

"I can't believe how critical I've become. I argue with people inside my head. My husband is a surgeon. We have lovely children. But since the miscarriage and the tubal ligation I had right afterwards, I haven't been able to get rid of the sadness. It makes me weepy even to talk about it. My sexual energy has been mostly dead. I even withdrew from my friends after I lost the baby. They had little kids and I couldn't bear being around their families. I made all kinds of excuses to isolate myself. I still want to be alone most of the time.

"I've been on lithium for ten years. My psychiatrist recommended that I try going off of it, but I quickly entered into another manic state. When I become manic, I believe that I'm carrying a very special baby who will save the world. I don't eat or sleep when I have one of those episodes, and my mind races. One time I received communication that one of my daughter's classmates, who was seriously ill, died. When I feel that way, I have a heightened awareness that I'm God's very special child, whom he loves more than anyone else. It feels as if something extremely important is about to take place. Everything happens so fast during those times. It's almost like I'm on a train taking us to a destination where there will be only goodness and peace. I sense that I have a role in enabling God's plan to unfold so that the world can become a better place. There's a feeling of urgency about it all. Even when I'm not manic I believe there's a divine plan.

"As a little girl, my feelings were very tender. My face would turn beet red when I felt embarrassed. I'd run upstairs to my room, throw myself facedown on the bed and go to sleep.

162

Overreacting was ingrained in me by my mother who taught me: 'Nobody loves me, everybody hates me, I'm gonna go eat worms.' I'm still a lot the same way.

"My first manic episode came six months after a severe depression. I had graduated from college and broken up with my boyfriend. I'd just begun working as a respiratory therapist at a busy hospital. I used a number of recreational drugs. Then I got so depressed that I ended up on a psychiatric ward for a month. They gave me Thorazine and Stelazine.

"Then I went to a contemplative Buddhist community. I became engaged and got married. We had two great kids. Then came the miscarriage. Shortly afterwards I went to India and spent time with some of the Tibetan refugees who had been tortured by the Chinese. I missed my sleep and it was very stressful. Fearing that someone would harm me and that I would never see my family again, I had another period of mania and was hospitalized.

"This year has been a roller coaster. High to low, up and down. I'd like to be myself again." Normally a good listener with a gentle temperament, Lily had a preference for solitude. She loved being by the ocean. Despite the fact that her husband was a physician, the fear of poverty was present, as was a fear of being alone and not being able to handle her life. Since childhood Lily had dreaded walking through the woods, fearing she'd come upon a snake. She was unable to remember any of her dreams. Her only physical complaint was intermittent constipation.

Sepia has benefited Lily to a remarkable degree. The prescription was based on her inability to find joy in her life, the history of sadness and loss of sexual energy following the miscarriage, of her dissatisfaction with and heightened degree of criticism of her family and her fear of poverty and snakes. Within days of taking the first dose, she reported feeling more of a cohesiveness in her thinking process. She experienced an immediate sense of lightness and happiness, as well as more energy and an increased capacity to accomplish her daily tasks. She decided to pursue additional training in respiratory therapy and switched to another hospital, which she enjoyed more.

"My husband and I are resolving some issues in our marriage. A channel of communication was opened which was previously unavailable. I'm finding myself going around the house imagining which wallpaper and pictures I want where. I even bought a new rug. I'm enjoying my home much more. There's also been a positive shift in my relationship with my son. I can feel my sexuality emerging in a variety of areas. I've lost ten pounds. Everyone notices the changes in me. I feel more connected to myself since taking the medicine. I'm simply not as caught up in the details of life as I was before."

Nine months after the initial dose of *Sepia*, Lily began to experience "a bit of an episode", which made her feel "about two feet off the ground". Her psychiatrist put her on Navane, an anti-psychotic medication, and Cogentin, to counteract the side effects of the Navane. We also repeated the *Sepia*. She soon felt significantly better and was able to discontinue the new medications after one week, although she had continued to take the lithium, which she had been taking all along. Lily explained, "This episode was so different from the others. I didn't lose it completely and I continued to work."

When Lily called a couple of months ago complaining of a debilitating flu, she said her throat felt as if it were closing, her temples ached, her face was hot and flushed and her sinuses were dry. Her body ached — particularly her neck and shoulders — her stomach was upset and her thirst was much less than usual. Since homeopathic medicine is also highly effective for most acute illnesses, we prescribed *Gelsemium* (yellow jasmine), which follows *Sepia* well. The *Gelsemium* "worked like a charm". Though Lily felt worse for an hour, she slept peacefully all night and woke up the next morning feeling quite well and able to go to work.

Lily is still taking lithium carbonate. Since beginning homeopathic treatment two years ago she has had only minor manic episodes, no severe or extended periods of depression and no hospitalizations. When we spoke to her recently, she told us that she felt 80% better overall than she did prior to homeopathy.

She continues to experience intermittent feelings of darkness, but nothing like the drastic ups and downs and constant sadness that was common previously. We anticipate that Lily will feel even better over time. She may or may not need to continue taking lithium for life. What is most important is that she feels a sense of happiness, direction and connection with life.

"My Clarity Disintegrated"

Joyce, a thirty-three-year-old woman from upstate New York, was at loose ends when we first spoke with her. "I don't know where to start. A lot of my situation comes from being mentally ill last summer. It's hard to talk about because a lot of it doesn't make sense and is hard to remember. I don't like the term 'mental illness'. When I was about fourteen I had anxiety, depression and trouble sleeping. I got really scared of everything. I worried about nuclear war and didn't want to talk much or be with friends. These same symptoms recurred every year from ninth through twelfth grade. I became hyper that year and was expelled from school. I was completely distraught that I didn't graduate from high school and I felt like a failure. At the same time, I went to live with my boyfriend, became pregnant and had an abortion after which I passed huge blood clots. Then I became really psychotic. I was sent to the psychiatric wards of three different hospitals. They gave me Haldol and a lot of other drugs." It was clear that her psychiatrists at this point diagnosed Joyce with schizophrenia.

"My clear thinking disintegrated. I became very scared and paranoid. Unable to sleep, I became extremely agitated and terrified. I read about a soccer game in South America at which some people were trampled to death and felt convinced that my sister was one of them. It wasn't true. I was on the locked psychiatric ward. While there, I had really weird religious thoughts and believed every meal on the psychiatric ward was the Last Supper. They gave me Haldol, Thorazine, Cogentin and Vivactil. A girl on the ward told me they were medicating me too much and told me to give my pills to her, so I did. After three weeks they transferred me to an adolescent ward. I remember being strapped down when I couldn't sleep one night. I threw myself onto the floor, distraught and confused. When they gave me my medications, I was convinced they were poisoning me. They finally took me off all the drugs."

Joyce continued to feel very depressed for quite a few months afterward. Living with her father, she returned to school to become an interior decorator. Four months after completing the course, she again decompensated. Diagnosed now with bipolar disorder, she was given lithium. When one of her instructors propositioned her, she again became psychotic. Able to avoid hospitalization, she existed marginally and never finished her studies. A few years later she experienced another manic episode.

"I did pretty well until a year ago. I was living with a friend and getting my bills paid. Then I moved in with my boyfriend. I went to art school but had a hard time staying focused. I drank coffee, smoked and went out dancing. It was like it happened overnight, right after my final exam. I had been getting kind of hyper but I hadn't noticed it. I tried to finish that last paper. I made my note cards but I couldn't get it together to write. I didn't sleep much that night.

"I started feeling hostile, mean, upset, unfocused. People told me that I needed help but I didn't think there was anything wrong with me. I alienated all of my friends. I stayed in that strange state for months. I drank a lot of alcohol. I destroyed my life. I blew all of my savings. I bought a boat but had nowhere to put it. I left my job, took all of my things and drove to Florida for two weeks, I charged it all to my credit card.

"My behavior was irrational. I threw out all of my clothes and burned all of my papers from the past. I flew to the Caribbean. The credit card company demanded that I raise my credit limit and so I did without even a second thought. I bought a three-hundred-dollar beaded sweater, a fifteen-hundred-dollar leather jacket with a mink lining and expensive jewelry. I slept with men. I'd never have done that kind of thing before. Then I went bankrupt."

166

During the six months prior to our first seeing Joyce she crashed. After another pregnancy and abortion she lost her car, subsisted on food stamps and barely functioned. She did not take her lithium. Lonely and confused, she felt as if she were dying. To no one's surprise, Joyce ended up back in the hospital but could only afford to stay there for one night because she didn't have health insurance. She was now working for a drapery company but mostly depended on her parents for money.

Joyce hadn't had a period since her last abortion, six months earlier. From all the trials she had endured, she looked at least forty. Her facial hair and body hair had become much thicker and she complained of long-standing psoriasis. She leaked after urinating, suffered from recurrent vaginal infections and her digestion was a mess. She felt weak, as if she had lost all of her muscle tone. She described her mental state as "in a fog" and "hanging on by a thread".

The medicine that helped Joyce was *Lilium tigrinum* (tiger lily). It is predominately for women with hormonal problems who have a wild feeling inside and frequently a conflict between their spiritual and sexual natures. One month after beginning treatment, Joyce's moods began to improve, as did her sleep. At the same time, she had begun taking Paxil and Depakote, which, she complained, caused hair loss. Her periods had not returned. Although Joyce was in much better shape than at the previous interview, we couldn't assess whether the improvement was due to the homeopathy or the psychiatric medications.

Six weeks later, her anxiety was gone and her night sweats (which she had not previously mentioned) had almost stopped. She no longer awakened feeling panicky. The psoriasis was under control. "I still want to have periods [she had not yet menstruated since her last abortion]. Work is going well. I am getting along with people." We were still not sure to what to attribute the improvement but were very happy that Joyce felt so much better. If the homeopathic medicine was working, we knew her periods would soon return, which they did after two more months. Her psychiatrist had advised her to discontinue the Depakote at that time, but she was still taking 20 milligrams of Paxil each day.

Seven months after beginning the *Lilium tigrinum*, Joyce reported feeling much better overall. She had experienced four normal periods, her digestion had improved, her emotions were on an even keel and work was going well. She described herself as neither depressed nor destitute. Under the guidance of her psychiatrist, she was gradually tapering off the Paxil.

At this point Joyce discontinued treatment and we have not seen her again. We include this case not because her treatment is complete, but because she describes the bipolar experience in such a real and candid way, because *Lilium tigrinum* can be very effective for bipolar disorder and to illustrate how effectively homeopathic and psychiatric medications can work together. One of the main challenges in treating patients with serious mental problems such as bipolar disorder is the lack of long-term follow-through with treatment.

22 Everything in Its Place

The Torment of Obsessive-Compulsive Disorder

On a day-to-day basis, life is a myriad of details. We get up when the alarm goes off, brush our teeth, bathe, get dressed, eat breakfast, feed our pets and get the kids off for school. Change the diapers, take out the garbage, return phone calls, check faxes and e-mail, and race out the door. This litany of events may take an hour or two, or longer.

What if you had to spend two or three times as long on each of these tasks in order to feel comfortable to move on to the next? Check the burner three times to make sure it was really turned off, go around twice to every door of your house to double-check the locks, wash your hands twenty times or do the laundry twice to eradicate every last germ, write and rewrite every note or letter four times to eliminate any possible mistake, ask your son over and over where he's going after school because you're so worried that something might happen to him? Iron and re-iron, fold and refold, lock, unlock and relock. The list is endless.

This is your plight if you suffer from obsessive-compulsive disorder (OCD). Regardless of where the attention and worrying are focused, the story is the same. It is one of terrific distress and obsession. Lives of constant checking and rechecking are excessive and exhausting. Howard Hughes, who from childhood was obsessed with avoiding germs, devised a system of "insulations" made from paper towels and tissues. Mr. Hughes insisted that doors and windows be sealed in order to prevent any germs from creeping into his house. (Sasson, et al., p. 7) A simple superstition such as "Step on a crack and break your mother's back" can lead to extremes, such as in the case of Dr. Samuel Johnson, an eighteenth century writer, who avoided any and all cracks between paving stones, "made extraordinary gestures or antics with his hands when passing over the threshold of a door", and touched every single post he passed

169

during his walks, going back if he happened to miss one. (Sasson, et al., p. 7)

Logic is beyond the point in OCD. You may know very well that your obsessions and compulsions do not make sense but feel compelled to carry them out anyway. Your urges may lead you to collect endless objects, sometimes until rooms are literally filled with boxes, piles of newspapers or magazines, or whatever else you have hoarded obsessively for fear of getting rid of anything. You may have to repeat certain rituals day after day — such as taking the same route to work or buying groceries in precisely the same order week after week — or to count incessantly or repeat certain actions a particular number of times. You may be so obsessed with the fear that someone may break into your home if every single window and door are not locked that you may be unwilling and unable to leave the house, which is called agoraphobia. In this way, OCD and phobias are sometimes interwoven. Pathological gambling, pulling out one's hair or eyelashes or other self-abusive habits, kleptomania, sexual obsessions and compulsions, extreme hypo-chondriasis, uncontrollable impulsivity, eating disorders and obsessive jealousy can all be manifestations of OCD.

The bottom line with OCD is that you are trapped in an imaginary prison for which only you have the key. You cannot rest until you have fulfilled your compulsions and, even so, your mind remains cluttered with obsessions. The media offered a poignant and insightful glimpse into the suffering of OCD through the character played by Jack Nicholson in the movie *As Good As It Gets*. As much as he wanted to engage in any degree of normalcy, it was impossible due to his quirks, fixations and fears. With OCD, tapes of routine events that have long passed may run endlessly in your mind. Tragic past events may become frozen in time, such as happened to Barbara, described in chapter 12, who had lost her daughter and was tormented by one obsession after another until receiving homeopathic treatment. There is no peace. Life becomes a series of rituals, impulses and rote, repeated actions with little room for spontaneity.

"I've Organized My Life around Protecting My Children"

It was her persistent headaches that led Arlene, a forty-year-old part-time receptionist from Philadelphia, to homeopathy. "I've had them since I was a teenager. They're full-blown migraines with nausea and dizziness. The only thing that helps is to vomit. Lately I've been getting them often and they last for four to five days at a time." We noticed that Arlene's hands fidgeted as she spoke. We doubted if it was a coincidence that she loved to sew and do needlework. It probably kept her hands busy. So did playing the piano and the autoharp.

"I've had bladder infections since I was a little girl. Now it's mainly spasms in my bladder. I haven't actually had an infection for several years. When I feel it starting to become sensitive, I start drinking lots of water and cranberry juice and put a hot water bottle on my lower abdomen. It seems to take care of the problem.

"I have two boys and two girls ranging in age from eight to eighteen. They're wonderful children. They don't seem to cause heartache like some people's kids. I'm very lucky that both of my parents are alive. My family is the most important thing in my life. I spend a lot of time chauffeuring around the kids from place to place. My mother and older brother have had some serious health problems during the last year, so I've been there for them. My aunt died of breast cancer last year. She was a very special person.

"I tend to be rather quiet, reserved and restrained. I'm a better listener than a talker. I have certain expectations of myself around other people. I make sure that I don't lose control around others. When my children come home late I worry a lot but I don't let them know that I feel out of control. It all goes back to when my oldest daughter was just a few months old. We were living in New York at the time. She and I were driving alone to visit my husband's family in Connecticut and took a break at a rest stop. It was late and ours was the only car there. I took the baby with me to the bathroom. Then I noticed a man standing around with his pants unzipped, masturbating. When the state trooper came, I was too afraid to get out of the car to speak with him. The man could have hit me over the head and kidnapped my baby.

"That event paralyzed me for a number of years. Since that moment I've been overprotective of my children. Before then I biked everywhere and walked alone. I had taken self-defense courses and didn't worry about getting attacked. Afterwards I became obsessed with the thought that he could have taken her from me. I didn't leave the house for a couple of months. I was totally aware of where everyone close to me was at all times. I still am. When a man looks at my daughters in a sexual way, I watch closely.

"I've organized my life around protecting my daughters. My husband and I try to be home before the children. As soon as I get home with the kids, I turn on all the lights and check behind all the doors before I let the kids come in the house. It used to be that I would wake up from the least little noise.

"How easy it is to drop that antenna that lets you pick up on any danger from the outside. I blamed myself for what happened that night. Rest stops were off limits for many years after that incident. We make sure that the kids don't go anywhere by themselves. They have a buddy system. I also worry about my husband or myself or one of my kids dying or something awful happening. Again it's the unknown that terrifies me. My dreams are weird. I see someone getting hit or strange people doing strange things. About once a month I wake up from a dream feeling threatened and grab on to my husband.

"I don't do well with bombastic, aggressive people who hit you in the face with their personalities. They make me feel like I have to put up my defenses so whatever they say won't affect me."

We knew that with the right homeopathic medicine not only would Arlene's headaches and bladder spasms improve but she would feel less vigilant and overprotective. *Kali bromatum* (potassium bromate) is a medicine for family-oriented people who feel tremendous guilt about something they have done or have failed to do. There is also a strong tendency among these people to have restless hands.

Arlene reported six weeks after taking the *Kali bromatum* that she felt considerably better overall. "Much better. I don't feel like I'm walking through a fog anymore. I'm much more with it mentally. Every once in a while I get a mild headache or bladder sensitivity but they clear up quickly and go away on their own. I don't get as flustered. My dreams are much calmer. I'm not waking in the middle of the night from violent nightmares anymore. My oldest daughter is going to Washington, D.C., with her choir. It scares me but I'm going to let her go. I'm handling it much better. That's a big step for me.

"My kids say I'm not hounding them so much. I'm beginning to realize that they need to make their own choices and decisions. It's amazing that I no longer worry about awful things happening. I think all of the anger from that night years ago is lessening. My anger toward men has diminished. I used to think that if I made love, I'd suffer the consequences and my bladder would hurt. I've let go of that notion and it feels much better. A whole new world has opened up for me."

Arlene has needed a total of three doses of the *Kali bromatum* over the past two and a half years that we have treated her. She continues to feel clear and calm. Her headaches are mild, few and far between. The bladder sensitivity has not recurred. Arlene does not feel as vulnerable to bombastic men. Her mental fog has not returned nor does she have the violent dreams. She continues giving her children more choices and freedom. "Not the paranoia I used to feel. This is the new me. I just don't feel panicky anymore when they're out of my sight."

A Passion for Baseball

We began treating Danny, an eight-year-old youngster from Florida, two years and four months ago. His mother explained that he seemed to view life differently from other children and was unusually full of energy. "Danny was an extremely temperamental, touchy infant. He didn't like to be held but was an insatiable nurser. We just couldn't find a way to settle him down before midnight. He's never exhibited signs of being tired like other kids. I'd wanted to become pregnant since I was a teenager but it wasn't happening. Every time my period arrived, I grieved. We finally conceived Danny through artificial insemination.

"He's a very sensitive child. The least little thing annoys him, such as odors or what people do or say. It all offends him and he becomes irritable and defensive. Danny's quite obsessive. He's very particular and literal. Everything has to be black or white. You have to place things in a certain way or he'll move them. Everything on his dresser has to be in a certain spot. If he sits with you on the sofa and your elbow touches his, he looks at you as if he'd hit you. He's very precise with rules of grammar and directions. If he's into pears, it's pears for breakfast, lunch and dinner. When I bought a new kind of cereal, he ate four bowls in a row, then wanted it every day. He'd bounce a ball all day long. He threw himself into pirates before, now it's sports. His goal is to go to every baseball park in the United States. Tics come and go. Coughing every two seconds, touching his eyes, asking questions over and over, double-checking things.

"New, exciting things are stimulating for Danny, although transitions are hard for him. He doesn't have a lot of common sense. The teacher says he's quite distractible in class. Novelty and excitement help him focus. At three he'd have to get up and pace across the room to focus before he could talk. He'd bounce, fidget and interrupt. Danny's intense!

"Things affect him deeply. Saying good-byes devastates him. Reading a book can make him very sad when he realizes that the characters aren't real and that he'll never meet them in person. His emotions are very close to the surface. He's a passionate kid. I'm very sensitive and was a lot like him as a kid. I think the obsessiveness comes from his dad."

Danny had a remarkable memory and loved to travel. His parents had tried Ritalin, Cylert and Prozac. Even the smallest dose of Ritalin made him frantic, weepy and kept him up until 2 A.M. Prozac took away his initiative and zest.

Medorrhinum (a nosode) helped Danny somewhat over a number of months, but we weren't satisfied with the degree of improvement. After seven and a half months, we changed his prescription to *Carcinosin* (another nosode), which made a significant difference for the better. His mother told us at the two-month follow-up appointment that Danny seemed to be less stuck in his thought process. He had less of a tendency to do or say the same thing over and over, and he also seemed more reasonable. Knowing that improvement from OCD can be slow, we decided to give the process more time without changing to another medicine.

After another five weeks, Danny's mother admitted that his obsessiveness had lessened by about 70 to 80%. Less excitable and overemotional, he was also interrupting less and his temperament was more even. His teachers observed a definite improvement from the OCD. Danny's teacher reported eight months after Danny started taking the *Carcinosin* that he had had a great year. More aware of others around him, he was not loud or inappropriate as he had been before; he was listening more and interrupting less.

The OCD continued to lessen significantly, but Danny became gloomy and fearful, especially about robbers. He even had a nightmare about a man coming into his house with a big chain saw. His focus diminished slightly. Danny had become much more social and empathetic, was very thirsty for cold drinks and didn't like spicy food. These symptoms matched indications for the medicine *Phosphorus*, a medicine that shares many symptoms with *Carcinosin*.

Danny's mom called a month later to report that his hopelessness and fears were much reduced. His fear of someone breaking in was about 80% less and he was taking things much less literally. Overall, she felt, he was 90% better. It has been two and a half years since we first treated Danny, and he continues to make excellent progress.

"She Came Out of Her Cocoon"

Wendy, a sixteen-year-old from Colorado, was a patient whom we treated through telephone consultations because there were no experienced homeopaths in her area. Her mother provided the following information: "Wendy's very bright, very nice, but a bit immature. She doesn't miss a beat. Take her into a room and she can remember every object on every wall. Wendy dances to her own drum. She's had to. Due to her tics, the kids picked on her terribly. It's taken a lot of courage for her not to follow the crowd.

"At the same time I discovered that I was pregnant with Wendy, I was told I had a lump in my breast. It turned out to be benign but it really gave me a scare. My mother's dog had to be put to sleep and she was out of her mind with grief. They buried the dog in our yard against my wishes. The combination of the dog and the breast lump made me extremely distressed. I became nauseous and threw up right up till I gave birth. Wendy was a gorgeous baby. I was terrified by her severe reaction to a DPT [diptheria-pertussis-tetanus immunization] shot. She cried for many hours and passed strings of pus from her rectum. They gave her antibiotic after antibiotic. It turned out to be an anal fistula. At seven months she began to show some jerking and eye rolling. Then came seizures. Again one anticonvulsant after another. I still wonder if it had anything to do with the DPT immunization.

"I started reading about learning disabilities. At first it didn't make sense to me because Wendy was so smart and seemed happy. The fistula returned and she had surgery at the age of nine. Soon after she started in a private school for kids with learning problems, she was teaching the other children. We moved her to a public school where she was teased unmercifully. The teachers wanted to put her in a special education program. We refused. She quickly moved from a remedial class to a

176

normal one that she made the honor roll in an accelerated class. However, Wendy's handwriting was an illegible scrawl."

This is a fearful kid. "She's petrified of moths and butterflies. Once, when she was very little, she remembers being scared by one. Wendy thinks they're horrible even if they're actually beautiful. If one is flying near her, she'll blink her eyes and flail her arms. She'll cringe even if she sees a tiny picture of them. Sleeping in her room would be out of the question if there was a moth inside. Of course she doesn't like to go to school because the kids tease her and she has no friends. She's very overweight and can act quite a bit younger than her age. A couple of years ago a boy pulled a knife on her, but she was afraid to tell us about it.

"Wendy's a jovial type, a happy kid. She only wants to do what she likes. Pizza and potatoes are about all she'll eat. When Wendy wants something, she'll bug me for hours. If she doesn't get her way, she'll ruin everything for all of us. But there's not a mean bone in her body. Justice is a big thing for Wendy. If she believes something is not right, she demands that something be done about it. Upon watching the news on television about people killing each other, she commented, 'People are so unkind.'" Yet Wendy could be oblivious to others' needs, is defensive and unforgiving.

"My daughter exhibited many different tics and compulsive habits. Once she went to the bathroom every two minutes. There was a period of having to touch the door or her shoes three times, another of pulling out her hair to the point of creating a bald spot, and still another habit of being compelled to touch the back of her throat." The specific compulsions came and went, one replaced by another.

Wendy shared with us that her favorite activity was to go online and access the chat rooms. She adored the idea that a bunch of kids could talk about games in computer language. Wendy confirmed that she was very afraid of butterflies and moths. When we asked her why, she replied they were ugly and scary. Heights scared her. One other curious bit of information from her mom was that she had an odd perception of danger. Going out in the ocean was fine but riding in a car was not.

This was a very unusual girl needing an equally unusual homeopathic medicine. Given her exaggerated fear of moths and butterflies, we studied the latest information about the newly tested medicine *Butterfly*. We learned that it addressed issues of feeling unprotected and unsafe, and we prescribed it. Anytime a homeopath gives a medicine — particularly a new one — for the first time, we take a pioneering step into the future of homeopathy. Even though the indications were preliminary, they seemed to fit Wendy.

We didn't speak to Wendy and her mom for four months. The first change, which occurred within forty-eight hours of taking *Butterfly*, was her willingness to play a computer game featuring a moth. Then Wendy became less anxious, more able to focus and talk, and her handwriting improved. Summer school went quite well. The tics decreased at least 70% and the overall improvement was at least 75%. Wendy seemed more mature and her eye contact was more appropriate. At a recent meeting with her teachers, they couldn't understand how she could have changed so much for the better. Once a moth flew so close to Wendy on a moonlit night that it practically touched her and she showed no fear.

Seven months after we first treated her, Wendy had put herself on a sensible diet, begun to exercise and was fitting comfortably into pants three sizes smaller. She had set a goal of losing a certain number of pounds within six months. Much more motivated, Wendy was looking forward to college and planning to major in Chinese. The tics were still dramatically reduced and the eye contact still very good. The only thing that had taken a turn for the worse was Wendy's handwriting. But with everything else progressing so nicely, it wasn't a big issue.

We have given Wendy infrequent doses of *Butterfly*. She has lost fifty pounds over the past six months and plans to lose forty pounds more. There has been quite a transformation. Her therapist calls it a miracle and wants Wendy's mom to share her experience with homeopathy with some of her other clients. Wendy is teaching herself Chinese in anticipation of college. She enjoys taking long walks every morning and was very excited recently when a fellow student actually offered her a ride. "Butterflies come out of their cocoons," exclaimed her mom, "and so has Wendy."

We recently had an opportunity to meet Wendy in person. She was quite happy about her progress and will begin attending a community college next month. Although her fear of butterflies and moths comes and goes, Wendy's self-esteem and social skills as well as her physical complaints have improved dramatically.

"The Monster Thing, That's Him"

Mickey, seven years old, was a friendly and charming boy. Since his parents lived across the country, we were unable to meet him personally, but his mother sent us a videotape of Mickey. She described him as extremely sensitive. "You can break his heart in two seconds. Like when he tries to make friends and can't. He almost collapses if you tell him he made a mistake. Mickey's not an aggressive child. Even though he has a blue belt in karate, he wouldn't even push another kid. One psychologist called him a loner. He only has one friend in school. When school first began, the other kids used to beat up Mickey every single day. A kid kicked him in the mouth and two of his teeth, which were already loose, came out. Mickey talks to himself, even when he's talking to others. Rejection and hurt are his constant companions. When he introduces himself to other kids, they tell him to go away.

"The monster thing, that's him. My son talks about monsters all the time — about the blood coming out. At the beginning he used scary stories to defend himself. The school complained that some of his classmates were having trouble sleeping because of his stories. Mickey's very creative. His stories either have no ending or someone dies. Like 'It was dark. A boy was walking through the forest. He found an alien's house. A big hand came out with lots of arms. The alien spat poison at the boy and he died.' He loves to learn poems, but only the scary ones.

"They diagnosed Mickey with OCD. He picks at his arms till he sees blood. There's cutting in his stories. He really likes Dracula and he's fascinated with the idea of drinking blood. At two he insisted on dressing like a vampire for Halloween and he wore that costume often afterwards. He tells me his stories while I'm driving. When I get out to fill the tank with gas, he doesn't even notice. When I get back in, he's still talking.

"Mickey has an obsession about germs. If someone coughs, he'll leave the room. He would never let you touch his food. He washes his hands frequently and brushes his teeth several times a day so he won't get cavities. Germs are a frequent topic of conversation. When I tell him I love him, he makes me repeat it several times. Mickey gets attached to rituals.

"He fears the dark, ants, losing me and the endings of his own stories. His father travels a lot for business and if I go outside, he runs to protect me. If a dog comes, he'll hide, and he's worried that something bad will happen. Mickey comes into bed with us every night.

"This child was slow to develop. Almost passive as a baby, he rarely cried. At one year he had the fine motor skills of a three-month-old. He couldn't even grab a raisin. Walking started at fifteen months. Mickey still doesn't catch well. He attends a school for children with learning disabilities. His language is at tenth-grade level, but his writing is very disorganized and dyslexic."

Mickey had a history of asthma, bronchitis and ear infections. He complained often of feeling tired. He had been diagnosed, by several psychiatrists and psychologists, with OCD, Asperger's syndrome and bipolar disorder. One prominent psychologist concluded that he had the profile of a serial killer.

To us as homeopaths, Mickey was one of the most unique and interesting children we had ever come across. This was a sweet, gentle child obsessed with thoughts of violence and blood. Even when persecuted by the other children, he didn't even strike back. He worried that something terrible would happen, yet talked incessantly about horror. We gave this sensitive child *China officinalis* (Peruvian bark) with very positive results.

Mickey's mom called us eight weeks after he took the *China*. "He became wired for a few days, then four days later started reading like he never had before. After six days he grabbed a piece of paper and wrote down fast and furiously three pages of karate techniques. His teacher asked him to read a book and he read ten. The monster thing is much less. When his sister asked him to read a book to her, he picked up Dr. Seuss. Before, it would have been a horror story. His father and I can't believe the incredible change in him."

Two months later Mickey's mom reported that his reading skills at present compared with before were like day and night. There was no talk of blood and he no longer picked at his arm. Not only did Mickey's teacher say that she saw absolutely no learning disability in him but he was nominated for an all-school award. Mickey still dreamed about monsters and scary creatures.

At our most recent appointment with Mickey, three months ago and two years after he began homeopathy, the only complaint was diarrhea following a vacation in Guatemala with his parents. His conversation was much more appropriate. Mickey's interests had expanded beyond monsters. He now loved basketball and planned to become a great basketball player. He also hoped to become an actor and a writer. He has been mainstreamed in school and is in classes with all gifted children. The teacher says he's one of her best students. Kids call to ask him to help them with their homework. He's the first to offer help to those in need. Mickey says he'll never say anything to hurt someone else no matter how rude they are. A serial killer? No way.

23 A Separate Reality

The Disorientation and Confusion of Schizophrenia

"It used to be called insanity. One day the world starts to seem distorted, too changeable, disjointed. There are voices speaking in your head telling you to do strange things. You feel driven by weird compulsions. You see objects, even people, that nobody else sees. You feel persecuted. You believe that your neighbors are controlling you with magnetic waves; people on television are manipulating you with subliminal messages; devils want to torture you.... Your head is full of chaos. Your sense of self has shattered into pieces." (Leviton, p. 42) This is the tormenting world of schizophrenia from which, far too often, there is no return.

Schizophrenia is probably the most debilitating of all mental illnesses. Characterized by recurrent acute psychotic episodes in which the person may experience hallucinations, delusions, confusion, a sense of disconnectedness from reality and, less frequently, violence and catatonia, it can be completely incapacitating. Withdrawn, socially isolated and cut off from normal relationships, livelihood and activities, many of these individuals are no longer capable of a full and rewarding life. Tragically, the illness often persists for life, depriving the individual of health and happiness. The best-case scenario for recovery is to intervene during the first psychotic episode, prior to hospitalization.

About 1% of the population of the United States suffers from schizophrenia and 2.5% of all health-care funds are allocated to these patients due to their periodic relapses, recurrent hospitalizations and decreased social and vocational functioning. (Amadio and Cross, p. 1149) Even more devastating to the individual and family is institutionalization, which occurs in 30% of these patients (Amadio and Cross, p. 1149), although in some cases it can bring relief to a burned-out family. At any given moment, about 100,000 schizophrenic patients languish in public mental hospitals. (Leviton, p. 42) The treatment in the United States is far more humane than chaining these unfortunate souls to their beds, as was routine in this country in earlier eras and still occurs in some developing countries.

In many cases conventional antipsychotic medications have only a partial effect. The person is still unable to lead a normal life. The compliance of schizophrenic patients in taking these medications is notoriously erratic due, in part, to their significant side effects, such as a shuffling gait, emotionless affect, trembling and a wry neck. Having observed many patients suffering from these sometimes irreversible repercussions of their well-intended medications is what led us to find a gentler, more effective solution.

We have had some successes, as you will see in the following cases. However, schizophrenia is definitely challenging to treat homeopathically and should only be attempted by a practitioner with considerable experience in both homeopathy and mental health. Even so, the results may be more limited than with other psychiatric diagnoses. As with conventional medicine, the longer the duration of psychosis before treatment and the greater the number of psychotic episodes experienced, the more guarded the prognosis. (Amadio and Cross, p. 1149) Another difficulty is making sure that the patient avoids exposure to coffee and the other factors that may interfere with homeopathic treatment. However, when treatment is successful, the rewards for the patient, family and homeopath are tremendous.

"I Must Be Doing It Wrong"

Gwen, a fifth-grade teacher, first came to us for homeopathic treatment fifteen years ago, complaining of chronic headaches, urinary incontinence, muscle twitching, restless legs and gas. She described herself as a passive person who avoided confrontations and went out of her way to please others. A thoughtful and highly principled woman, it was unusual for Gwen to stand up for her convictions. "I'm an eel. I move around things. If one thing doesn't work, I'll try another." Introspective and philosophical, Gwen had been a good child and was a good adult, trying to do what was expected of her.

Gwen's incontinence, muscle twitching, cystitis and headaches were reduced considerably from taking *Staphysagria* (stavesacre). Seven years into treatment, her complaints shifted to chronic hoarseness, throat clearing and severe, violent belching with gastric reflux. *Phosphorus* provided considerable relief.

Then a curious thing happened. We hadn't heard from Gwen for a year. At age fifty-six, she came back to see us confiding that she had suffered an acute psychotic episode, which had pushed her into another reality. "I wasn't cooking on all burners. I'm seeing a psychiatrist and he has me on Stelazine. He encouraged me to come back and see you. I'm having problems at the school where I teach. I don't have very good boundaries. People's stuff sticks to me. I say too much, give too much. I had a dream about a really solid foundation of floor, which needed a fire to keep it going. The plywood walls were separating from the solid tongue-and-groove floor."

Listening to Gwen speak, it was apparent that she was very hoarse again. Her terrible headaches had also returned. "The past few weeks there have been terrible excruciating pains in the head and neck."

We asked her more about her recent experience. "The principal in my school is a three-hundred-pound Asian woman. She's the maternal archetype. I try to withdraw from her. She demeaned me and I was terrified. She and another teacher in my school seemed to work together to make things hard for me, to cut me off from my job satisfaction and effectiveness. It caused me to feel more terror. My mouth was completely dry for a whole month. I felt adrenaline rushes and found it hard to focus my mind. I couldn't seem to get enough water.

"I was assigned a class that didn't want to learn. It felt like the principal did that by design. I began to think that the FBI was bugging my classroom. I was in utter agony. I couldn't go out in crowds. I thought people were watching me. It was hard to go out in public, to the grocery store. I thought my house was bugged, so I started writing notes to my husband. I felt demeaned, diminished. The meaning of my job was threatened." Gwen had been stressed to the point of suffering acute psychosis.

Stelazine broke Gwen's paranoid train of thought. She stayed on the drug for one month while she took medical leave from school. Due to the return of her incontinence, belching and hoarseness, and because Gwen desired salty food and fruit, we again gave her *Phosphorus*. This is a medicine for thirsty, sensitive, fearful yet compassionate people who pick up very easily on the thoughts and feelings of those around them.

Several months later Gwen again began to experience anxiety and terror at school. "I'm convinced that others are thinking about me. I'm trying to please people whenever I can." She had experienced another mild psychotic episode, which had kept her home from work for three days, and she was back on Stelazine.

At this point we asked Gwen what she felt was the theme that most bothered her throughout her life. "It's being the victim, the outcast. Separation from my family. I was the black sheep, the scapegoat, the schoolyard victim. I never felt part of the group. We moved a lot. I envied the people who had friends. My husband and I opposed the Vietnam war, leading my parents — conservative Republicans — to reject us. They refused to talk about our beliefs and lifestyle. The hardest thing in my whole life was the parental rejection and not being able to transcend it. I've felt extremely guilty that I couldn't give them what they wanted. You know, I'm a people pleaser.

"Last spring, during my psychotic break, I had a fear that I was being framed, imprisoned and condemned for being who I was and for what I was sharing with the children. I felt more and more threatened. I withdrew more and more. I felt shunned, excluded, as if I weren't teaching well."

We then prescribed *Zincum metallicum* (zinc) because of Gwen's feeling that she was a criminal and her past history of restless legs. She continued to do very well with infrequent repetitions of the medicine for the next three and a half years. During that time Gwen did experience two milder recurrences of her paranoid thinking, at which time she took the *Zincum* again, along with a brief regimen of low-dose Stelazine prescribed by her psychiatrist, who continued to be very supportive of her homeopathic treatment.

Gwen continued to feel stronger within herself, spending time in nature and creating beautiful watercolor paintings. In an effort to deeply understand herself and her circumstances even more, she worked intensively on dream analysis and gained many more profound insights into herself. In Gwen's words: "I'm doing quite well. I feel stronger and more solid, more mentally together. I am more willing to be courageous, to be myself again. I feel more connected spiritually and I can pray again. It's something I've really longed for. I am more in touch with my spirit and integrity."

At a more recent visit, Gwen shared, "I've felt really good, very centered and focused in the classroom, handling a million details. Before, I couldn't keep the thread together. One of my watercolor pieces was even accepted in a show. All the pieces are fitting together. I have my courage, self-respect and dignity back."

Eventually we fine-tuned Gwen's prescription a bit more. Given her successful response to *Phosphorus* in the past, we gave her *Zincum phosphoricum* in an attempt to help her with her persistent urinary incontinence. Gwen has felt even better overall and has needed very infrequent repetitions of the *Zincum phosphoricum* during the past seven months. Her incontinence has improved considerably. She has taken one five-milligram dose of Stelazine now and then when she has felt a lot of stress at school. She has never needed to be hospitalized. A patient for twenty-five years, Gwen has never had a recurrence of these symptoms, has had no need for psychiatric medications, and continues to see us periodically for general health concerns.

"I'm Terrified That I'll Hurt Others or They'll Hurt Me"

Freddie was a fifteen-year-old high school student from the Olympic Peninsula. His mother, a lobbyist for alternative medicine, was familiar with homeopathy and contacted us. Aware of the less-than-stellar long-term success of conventional medicine in treating schizophrenic patients, she hoped we could help her son. Freddie had suffered a psychotic breakdown two months earlier. When we saw Freddie for his initial appointment, he reminded us of a terrified deer paralyzed by the headlights at night on a forest road.

"I'm scared of everything. My hands might strangle me, so I sit on them so they won't get me. I used to hear voices about a month ago but I don't anymore. I've been afraid for a long time. It happened first when I was eight years old. For some strange reason, I just wanted to hurt everybody. Mostly strangers. I wanted to make them feel scared so they'd know what I was going through. I didn't tell my mom because I was embarrassed about thinking that way.

"I get afraid that the cabinets might fall or the chair might swallow me up. Sometimes I feel safe with my teacher at school but I don't go often because the other kids might hit me. I see pictures in my head of me getting hurt. My dreams move very fast. I usually get hurt and sometimes I hurt other people. Before I went on the drugs my psychiatrist gave me, I didn't know if my dreams were real.

"When I feel really frightened I like to write poems and stories. Fantasy stories about wizards or science fiction. It's very hard for me to go to school because I have to talk to people. I can't concentrate well and my mind keeps going back to those thoughts about injury. Sometimes the images are bloody, with body parts being thrown into a river."

Freddie's mother was understandably distraught. She had first noticed a change in Freddie eight months earlier. Previously adventurous and confident, Freddie had become quiet, sullen, gloomy and secretive. Drawn to the depths of his bedroom, he was absorbed for hours at the computer, where he wrote voraciously, carefully protecting his work from anyone's eyes. It was as if he were in some type of trance. The tone of Freddie's writing was dark — mostly poetry about death. Some of the poems, which recounted murders, were frighteningly macabre. Freddie produced reams of poems as his consciousness streamed onto paper. Over the previous year, according to his mother's report, Freddie had become more and more fascinated with mystery and horror novels, the science-fiction television program *The X-Files* and the paranormal.

Unable to sleep, the young man had become confused and melancholic. Freddie's high school personnel were alarmed by his behavior and suggested a referral to a children's psychiatric hospital. The first psychiatrist Freddie consulted prescribed Zoloft and Haldol. A second doctor replaced the Haldol with Risperdal. The Zoloft perked him up, and the Risperdal took away the hallucinations. The two physicians did not agree conclusively on a diagnosis. Possibly bipolar disorder, severe depression with psychosis or schizophrenia.

Without the medications, Freddie felt lethargic and unable to concentrate. Weepy and dazed, he could not make it through even a day at school. Upon his physician's advice, he had discontinued his medications one week prior to his first appointment with us.

Normally, in a case such as Freddie's, we would want the patient to continue with his psychiatric medications until we found an effective homeopathic medicine so as to avoid a decompensation and possible hospitalization.

Our impression of Freddie was that he was extremely bright, introspective, creative and sensitive. We thought it would be a terrible shame for such a brilliant individual to be trapped in a schizophrenic world for life. The medicine that took the edge off of Freddie's fears for a number of months was *Thea* (tea), a medicine for people who have an unexplainable desire to injure or kill others.

Freddie eventually shared with us his deep interest in physics. He loved to immerse himself in the theories of quantum mechanics and to surf the Web for the latest developments in physics. This fascination led us to prescribe for him the medicine *Hydrogen*. Patients who need this medicine are often extremely deep thinkers and highly sensitive individuals who search intently for the meaning of life. They may soar to blissful states in which they feel integrally connected to the universe, then plunge to the depths of despair and separation. These people often share a common interest in the stars, the planets, black holes and the farthest reaches of the universe.

During the twenty-six months we have treated him, Freddie has not needed any more antipsychotic medication. Nor has he been hospitalized. He has, however, had his ups and downs. He has benefited from *Hydrogen* for the past year, although his state has definitely fluctuated. On the positive side, he is attending school full-time, has gotten his driver's license, has been able to interact more socially with his peers and was recently hired for a summer job. His moods and thoughts continue to vacillate periodically, although he has continued to remain relatively stable and able to function, which may suggest the diagnosis of bipolar disorder rather than schizophrenia. At his recent visit, Freddie reported feeling "much more together", free of fears and "doing better in all ways". This is admittedly a case in progress rather than a cure. Freddie sometimes feels calm and secure but still has periods of anxiety and instability. We will need to continue to treat Freddie for at least two more years on a regular basis in order to assure that he continues to do well. It will be particularly important to follow him closely during the delicate period of graduating from high school, entering college and embarking upon the life of a young adult.

A Battle Between Good and Evil

Camilla first consulted us ten years ago. As a Christian missionary, God was the foundation of her life. Camilla began by telling us about an annoying, chronic eczema that

189

had bothered her since childhood. Treatments of all kinds, conventional and natural, proved unsuccessful. But eczema was the least of Camilla's problems. Her mental state interfered much more with her life and normal functioning.

While in South America on a missionary tour, Camilla had become uncommunicative shortly after breaking up with her boyfriend. Lacking self-confidence since childhood, the breakup proved more than Camilla could handle. Her mind became confused, her thoughts disconnected and her ideas abnormally rigid. Unable to find the correct words during conversations, she knew something was terribly wrong with her mind. The only thing that made her feel better was to compulsively clean and to serve other people. We noticed that her voice trailed off mid-sentence and that it was very difficult for her to remain on track while telling us her story.

Above all, Camilla felt an urgent challenge to decide between good and evil. Though desiring to become pure in the sight of God, she felt torn by sexual thoughts. Camilla was raised by very strict, self-righteous parents and had been made to feel that even thinking about sex was very wrong. This led to tremendous guilt on her part. She now felt a strong impulse to swear, which went against her very nature. It seemed strange that such a sweet, kind, sincere, religious woman would be tormented by such dark thoughts. We very much wanted to help her regain her peace.

Camilla needed homeopathic *Anacardium* (marking nut), a valuable medicine for individuals with low self-esteem who feel a tremendous inner conflict between good and evil. It is common for such a patient to describe an image of an angel on one shoulder and a devil on the other, each whispering instructions into her ear. In some cases the inner torment is so extreme as to result in malicious actions and violence. This was definitely not the case with Camilla. Her violence, expressed in the desire to curse, remained within, at least as far as we knew. *Anacardium* also happens to be an excellent medicine for eczema, a chronic problem for Camilla.

At last-minute notice, Camilla left on another missionary trip right after we treated her. We would have preferred that she remain close by and under as little stress as possible during the first two to three months of treatment. She next saw us three months after taking the medicine and reported feeling much clearer mentally. "I realize now that I felt in the middle of a battleground between good and evil. That's not the case anymore. I used to see God and Satan in everything. Not now." Camilla still had some desire to swear. The eczema on her hands and legs was gone but she still had some small eruptions under her right arm.

The *Anacardium* continued to allow Camilla to think clearly and her self-confidence became enhanced. The desire to swear diminished and her eczema improved considerably. Four months after taking the initial dose of the medicine, Camilla continued to function quite normally. We lost track of her when she returned to her missionary work in South America until she came in for another appointment eighteen months later. At that time she continued to feel happy and well.

"Love, Love, Love"

Although homeopathy can sometimes be immensely helpful in the treatment of schizophrenia, we do not intend to paint too rosy a picture. With conventional or alternative treatment, one of the major obstacles to cure is lack of compliance. Sometimes even when the correct medicine is found, the patient either sabotages or abandons treatment, as shown in the following case.

Twenty-five-year-old Paul, like Freddie, was brilliant and showed great promise. His mother, a writer from Maine, who was very satisfied with her own homeopathic treatment, asked if we could treat Paul for schizophrenia. We agreed to do our best. His mother explained, "As early as the fifth grade he began to run around with the wrong type of kids, and it never stopped. Extremely sensitive, he played hockey but never had a taste for the killer and aggressive instinct necessary to be a great player.

Harmony was extremely important to Paul." Friction and discord were to be avoided at all costs. In fact, when Paul's mother reprimanded his siblings, Paul would tell her, "Love, love, love".

Paul began to abuse drugs and alcohol at age ten. His father had been a heavy drinker. His mother wondered whether he was affected by the Paregoric, an opiate-containing over-the-counter drug for treatment of diarrhoea, that he was given as a child. Paul never felt that his father was there for him. He was strongly affected by his parents' arguments and had difficulties around large groups of people.

Married at twenty, Paul then enrolled in a large university in the Northeast, where he made straight A's and the dean's list. His roller coaster between addiction and sobriety continued, causing strain to his marriage. At the age of twenty-two, Paul took LSD. This drug was not new to him, but around that same time his wife made a final break with him. The combination of stresses threw him into a psychotic state. He paced, felt paranoid and was unable to sleep. During the psychotic episode, Paul didn't eat, smoked constantly and talked nonstop nonsense. He developed a very heightened yearning for world peace, felt connected to another dimension and described feeling transparent. Whenever Paul was schizophrenic, he became vegetarian — at other times he ate meat — and lamented the animals that others ate, saying, "They cried when they died." Paul was disturbed by voices telling him to kill himself.

This was only the first of a series of psychotic episodes followed by hospitalization. In each case, Paul was given antipsychotic medications, took them for a while, discontinued them, then turned again to recreational drugs and alcohol. The pattern was yet unbroken when we first saw him. We felt quite optimistic about helping Paul turn his life around for good.

We questioned him in depth about his experiences with LSD because it seemed to be one of the causative factors that propelled him into psychosis. He explained that his LSD experiences during high school were pleasurable and produced a heightened sense of awareness. Other than hallucinating a couple of times, Paul felt pretty well. His brain became more awake, and he laughed for an hour at a time. However, the last LSD trip proved to be Paul's undoing. He felt agitated and anxious, over-stimulated as if his brain were over-firing and paranoid that others knew what was going on inside his brain. In an attempt to neutralize the over-stimulation, Paul turned again to alcohol.

At the time that we first saw him, Paul told us that he was blessed with a heightened ability to relate to others and was able to transmit thoughts without speaking. "Other people can hear what I'm thinking. My mind's totally open. I see others getting hurt and believe that I am the source of the negativity that creates their injuries and pain. If my body dies, then I can relieve their pain. But if I cut myself, I don't bleed to death. I know that because I've tried to kill myself a number of times.

"I prefer to be alone because I'm uncomfortable around most people. No matter what I do or where I am, I'm connected with a voice, an animal or a tree. I try to keep my thoughts lofty and positive, but it's terrifying. It's like there are two me's. One is a kind, loving individual. The other is negative and can't stop bad things from happening to others. Very rarely do I like the connection that I feel. It's easy to travel back and forth in time to the past or future. It's very hard for me to live in the moment because I'm constantly bombarded with things. There are no boundaries. I can do time travel and walk through walls. I wonder when others will wake up to the fact that they can, too."

To a homeopath, the more unique and unusual the symptoms, the better, so we found Paul to be fascinating. There happens to be a homeopathic medicine, *Anhalonium* (mescal cactus), made from a psychoactive Mexican plant, which, when ingested, induces symptoms very similar to Paul's. It is used for people, often with a history of hallucinogenic drug use, who feel completely merged with the world around them. They are generally kind, loving, open, compassionate individuals. The problem is that they are much too open and lack the boundaries needed to live in a world that is not necessarily filled with love, harmony and beauty. People like Paul are so sensitive and idealistic that they often resort to psychoactive drugs in order to make the world a livable environment.

Paul reported at his appointment one month later that everything was going better. "There is less chatter and activity in my mind. I feel more connected, relaxed, functional. After the treatment, the door between me and the world was shut, which was good. I was just about to lock it. Then after I drank coffee, the door reopened. I'm no longer traveling back and forth in time. It's almost like I have a different life. Now I understand that my ideas about time travel were a little wacky. Life is pleasurable now that I'm not communicating with other people and voices. Plus, my heartburn is completely gone."

We were very happy about Paul's response to the medicine and knew the *Anhalonium* could transform his life in a positive way. Unfortunately, he returned to drinking coffee, which interrupted his improvement, and later to drugs and alcohol. Although we urged him to give up his addictions and return to homeopathic treatment, he has not.

We continue to treat his mother and hear about Paul from time to time. He has never returned to a functional, happy, productive life. We hope that someday he is able to leave drugs and alcohol behind, because we feel sure that homeopathy could help him over the long run. This type of case is heartbreaking for us, but we need to remind ourselves that we must each decide for ourselves, for better or worse, how to lead our lives and which choices to make.

24 Painful Memories That Won't Quit

Surviving Sexual Abuse

When we first began working in the area of mental health in the mid- to late '70s, sexual abuse was rarely mentioned. As a psychiatric social worker in the emergency room of Harborview Medical Center, part of Judyth's job was to counsel women who were brought in by Rape Relief immediately after they were abused. However, the notion that childhood sexual abuse was commonplace never came up in her social-work training. Schizophrenia, depression, bipolar disorder, anxiety, borderline personality dis-order, alcoholism, drug abuse — but never childhood sexual abuse. It was only when we became homeopathic physicians and began to hear the appalling stories of so many women sexually abused during childhood that the prevalence began to sink in. There have been times when it was hard to keep from crying while hearing the terrible experiences these adults had had as children. Even more sobering was the persistent long-term damage often done to their relationships and self-image.

An estimated 114,000 cases of childhood sexual abuse were substantiated in 1994, with perhaps half to three quarters of these children receiving subsequent counseling. (Finkelhor and Berliner, p. 1408) Sexual abuse is an experience rather than an illness, but it can lead to other disorders such as depression, drug and alcohol abuse, anxiety, phobias, borderline personality disorder or dissociative identity disorder. Intimate relationships can be marred for life, generally due to a withdrawal and fear of intimacy or, less often, to an exaggerated sexual acting out. Particularly devastating are instances of gang rape and ritual abuse; however, any sexual abuse of any kind can have deep and permanent effects. The individual's trust in adults or parents may be shattered. Self-blame, either for not saying anything to anyone or for partially enjoying the attention and physical experience, is common. The result may be a perception of being dirty, disgusting, undesirable or at the least, very confused.

Conventional treatment, which can involve years of individual, family or group psychotherapy, benefits only some children who have been abused and has little effect on such problems as aggressiveness and sexualized behaviors. (Finkelhor and Berliner, p. 1415) Homeopathy can have a profound effect on the psyche of the sexually abused child or adult — even years later — and can enhance the effectiveness of other therapies significantly.

"They Did Awful Things to Me"

Carmen, age fifty, a computer programmer from Colombia, was referred to us by a friend of hers. She had been diagnosed eight years earlier with chronic fatigue syndrome and fibromyalgia. While she was ill, Carmen's weight skyrocketed from 135 to 300 pounds. Carmen also complained of severe constipation for which she took herbal laxatives.

"I feel very confused. Everything bothers me. My energy is terrible. I feel very anxious. Sometimes my mind just drifts off when I'm driving. I can feel as if I'm in a strange place and get disoriented about time. My memory is very poor. All of my symptoms — the chronic fatigue, fibromyalgia and the confusion — began with a flu eight years ago.

"I'm not a happy person. This is my second marriage. My first husband died. I was sexually abused before the age of five by my grandfather, then two of his friends. They did awful things to me. They even made me do something with a dog. I love dogs, but they bring back bad memories. When I see a dog humping, I feel sick.

"My mother wasn't married when I was born. I came out of the womb with severe eczema all over my body. She abandoned me. I was passed from relative to relative — the odd kid out. While the abuse was happening, I tried to run away. They tied me to a clothesline. There was no one around to protect me.

"I married soon out of high school and had a little boy. My husband was killed in a motorcycle accident. My mother didn't even come to the funeral. It's hard for me to be around people and I just want to be left alone. I feel guilty that people don't like me because they think I don't like them. Men make me feel very uncomfortable, especially big men.

"My life is a struggle. I am the breadwinner in our family and I resent it. I've worked since I was fifteen, and it's time that someone took care of me. I feel guilty about dredging up the past, but I haven't been able to get over what happened to me. They tied me by my wrists when they abused me. My arms and hands are still swollen and painful." The thought of sex with her husband was repulsive.

"I felt so dirty after they did all of those things to me. I've gone through years of psychotherapy and it's helped a lot; but I still have a long way to go." Carmen felt out of her body much of the time, as if she were floating. Then she would hear the words "get back in there," wake up, and slam back into her body again.

Carmen's story touched us deeply. The terrible indignities that she suffered as an innocent child can never be undone, but significant healing has allowed her to leave the past behind and move forward in a direction of healing. *Lac caninum* (dog's milk) is for people who feel they have been treated as the underdog, true or not. In Carmen's case, she was clearly treated as less than human. People who have experienced such derision, abuse and disrespect often feel that they must basically apologize for being alive, that they must be subservient in order to survive.

Six weeks after taking the *Lac caninum,* Carmen reported that her emotional state was a whole lot better. "I don't feel so stuck and I can see possibilities. My outlook isn't as negative and the confusion is much better. The disorientation is gone. I realize what a doormat I've been all of my life."

One year after she began the homeopathy, Carmen's confusion was still greatly diminished and her memory still greatly improved. She felt much less affected by her past and more comfortable around her dog. This is definitely a case that will need to be followed over time, but the medicine fits Carmen well; and given the terrible trauma to which she was subjected as a child, she has responded very favorably to the *Lac caninum*.

A Man with Sexual Guilt

George, a forty-year-old stockbroker from Oregon, was divorced three years before seeking homeopathic treatment. Mild and soft-spoken, his troubles started when his ex-wife invited him over for a visit. She wanted to make love, but he was reluctant because he no longer loved her. Against his better judgment, he gave in to her and regretted it ever since. During their lovemaking he sustained an abrasion on the shaft of his penis, which was very slow to heal. Fearing that he had contracted a yeast infection from their sexual contact, he applied soap, a topical antibiotic and a camphor-containing ointment topically to his penis. It became quite inflamed. Desperate to arrest what he assumed was an increasingly serious infection, he applied kerosene. His penis became quite red, sore and swollen. He consulted a dermatologist, who advised him to leave it alone and let it heal.

George felt quite embarrassed that he had injured himself and angry at himself for having made love to his ex-wife again. Depression followed and he began to doubt himself sexually. About this time he also developed urethritis, which was treated with anti-biotics. He sought therapy and tried to resolve the guilty feelings that continued to plague him. George began to feel good enough to begin a new relationship, which he was enjoying very much.

The inflammation of his penis was resolved except for a small, localized brownish spot. About eight months later, near the anniversary of his marriage to his ex-wife, George's penis and scrotum suddenly became bright red and inflamed, similar to a bad sunburn. Very worried, he saw numerous doctors and had many tests. The diagnoses were varied, including contact dermatitis, yeast allergy, seborrheic dermatitis and an allergic reaction to antibiotics. After four months the condition was resolved using topical tea compresses.

George again began to feel guilty about having had sex with his ex-wife. He obsessed over having caused injury to himself. He started psychotherapy again and began to avoid sex, fearing that his symptoms would return. Consumed with worry and self-blame, George also obsessed over never being normal again. Melancholic and moody, he was unable to enjoy sex anymore.

George had married at twenty-five and he and his wife had had a child; but the relationship began to go sour after his wife had an affair and left him. They got back together and had another child but eventually divorced, with shared custody of their two children. After the divorce, George felt lonely and a failure. He felt guilty for having relationships for "just sex", particularly regarding the last sexual encounter with his ex-wife. During his marriage, his wife hadn't wanted to have sex with him very often. Angry about having to ask for it and feeling pressured into having a child too early, he harbored resentment toward her. "She made me feel like there was something wrong with me." His anger turned inward, George did not even recognize that he was angry, much less identify the cause. His response was to blame himself for everything, whether or not he was responsible.

George felt resentment toward his birth father, who had abandoned him soon after he was born. Believing that his father didn't love him, he was not able to bond with his stepfather, either. Lonely as a teenager, George never quite fit in. He masturbated from an early age, more frequently during his teens, when he called it his "secret sin".

When asked about dreams, George related one about a "rat man" growing out of his groin from an embryo. This was related to a movie he had seen in which a man had to face his deep fear of rats. George's deepest fear was castration or genital mutilation.

George benefited from *Staphysagria*, which is helpful for quiet, refined men with genitourinary and skin problems who have a strong tendency toward self-blame, reproach and suppressed anger. George's repressed emotions wreaked havoc on his sexual organs.

At his six-week follow-up, George reported that the irritation on his scrotum had disappeared and he felt more stable emotionally. More able to express his anger toward his ex-wife, he also recounted a recent dream about releasing anger. His sexual energy had increased.

During a partial relapse of his symptoms three weeks later following dental work, George recovered a memory of being sexually abused at the age of four by an uncle. This was not too surprising because the extent of his physical and emotional emphasis on sex and the genitals from such an early age often suggests a history of childhood sexual abuse. At the same time, George also recalled that anger had not been permitted in his family and that whenever he outwardly expressed his anger his mother made him earn back her approval.

A year later, George was no longer having any problems with sex and did not feel guilty about the incident with his ex-wife. He had grown a lot in that year and was proud of how far he had come. Positive and more expressive, the relationship with his girlfriend continued to grow. He felt very good about his sexual life and had experienced only one minor episode of irritation of his penis.

Now, four years after beginning homeopathic treatment, George has needed six doses of the *Staphysagria*. He is happy working in a new office, has married his girlfriend and has a satisfying sex life. The sexual difficulties and genital symptoms are gone and he feels very confident and optimistic about his life.

"I Will Not Tolerate Rudeness"

Helen, a fifty-nine-year-old florist from Sacramento, had entered menopause six years earlier. Following a tubal ligation at thirty-five, her hormones had begun to decline noticeably.

A no-nonsense kind of woman, she told her story straight and to the point. "My medical doctor put me on hormone replacement for my hot flashes but I couldn't take the mood swings. I've been married for ten years. I wouldn't trade him for the world. It's my second marriage and I got a winner this time. My daughter is thirty and lives across the country.

"I like things organized. I get things done and get them done right. I'm not a procrastinator. I want things to work, and if they don't, I find out why. I'm here to find out about this menopause thing. The irritability is the worst part of it. I'll only go to an M.D. as a last resort because they go for the symptom rather than the cause of the problem. Figuring out what my body's telling me is what makes sense to me.

"Given a choice, I'd rather spend time with my husband. He watches too much television, but he pays the electric bill so I'll live with it. My temper can get hot. I can't handle being blamed for something that's not my fault, and most of all, I can't handle rudeness. I absolutely will not tolerate someone hurting another who is defenseless. You'd call me a protector. Kids used to call me stupid and dumb, but I never use those words.

"When I get really upset, I don't blow up or yell at a person; I keep it inside. Maybe act politely to that person but I'm not friendly and won't go out of my way for her. That's my way of handling anger. To cross them off and just act politely. I just won't stand for being treated rudely.

"My mother was the marshmallow in the family. Dad was the authority figure, who provided food, shelter and the necessities. The rest of the kids treated me like the outcast, the oddball. It made me mad because I never understood why I wasn't accepted. My parents were practical people. No special clothes. Nothing fancy.

"I married at twenty-three. Bad news. He had an affair with my best friend and never paid any attention to our daughter. I divorced him and moved two thousand miles away with my daughter. The hardest thing for me is dealing with my anger.

I even lose my temper with my loving husband. I guess it comes from being hurt and rejected a lot as a child. I felt like something was wrong with me. Peer pressure and insults are the worst thing." Helen's main physical problem was bloating and gas.

Helen told us from the very beginning that she was convinced we could help her and that she was committed to continuing with treatment until that happened. It's a good thing she had patience because it took nine months and six medicines to find the one that has helped Helen ever since. She had been seeing a psychotherapist for a number of years, with considerable benefit. Six months after we began to treat her, memories of sexual abuse by her grandfather started surfacing. Taken by surprise, she needed a number of months to sort it all out. She was finally able to remember the origin of her digestive problems and explained how she had to pull her knees up to her chest to get relief. That was our clue to prescribe *Colocynthis* (bitter apple), a medicine for sensitive people who respond to rudeness and insult with indignation and anger.

Helen felt significantly better after taking *Colocynthis* and has continued to feel better over the past year. Those who think homeo-pathy is only placebo need only look at a case like Helen's to realize that the good intentions of the homeopath are not enough to produce the degree of healing we are seeking for our patients. Although both Helen and we wanted to see rapid improvement, progress was not made until we found the right medicine for her. Upon her request, we also referred her to a different psychotherapist, who was able to help her with eye movement desensitization reprocessing (EMDR).

At present, a year and nine months after Helen first consulted us, she has scaled a mountain of repressed memories and emotions. Her gas is reduced and she feels much better emotionally. "Every once in a while my anger flares up for a few days; then I think about how I wish I would have handled it." Helen's marriage is going very well since her irritability has diminished greatly. She has worked through most of her feelings about the abuse and feels generally well. It is traumatic to realize that one has been sexually abused, at any age. We commend her for her courage and perseverance during the healing process.

25 A Case of Mistaken Identity

The Fragmented World of Dissociative Identity Disorder

Dissociative identity disorder (previously called multiple personality disorder) is a condition in which a person dissociates to such a degree that she leads two or more lives independently — usually alternately — each personality seemingly able to function separately. (Salama, p. 75). One personality at a time generally predominates while the others recede. Six thousand cases of dissociative identity disorder (DID) had been diagnosed in North America as of 1995 (Salama, p. 75), and since 1986, over seven hundred scientific articles, chapters and books have been published on the subject. There are four to seven women with DID for each man with the disorder. (Salama, p. 77). Suicidal thoughts are common in these people. Like sexual abuse, it has often been ignored in the past and can be very difficult to diagnose, even for a skilled and experienced physician, psychologist or psychotherapist.

One of the most likely events to trigger DID is childhood sexual abuse. The confused child cannot understand the experience, the relationship, and how he or she is supposed to respond. A common reaction to this dilemma is to dissociate or leave the body, to find a safe place to retreat, to literally go somewhere else. In this sense, DID is an understandable adaptation to the overwhelming trauma. It is a rather drastic attempt to integrate into one's consciousness an event or series of events that are too much for the normal psyche to bear. Physical escape may be impossible, so escape within the psyche appears to be the best or only choice. Years later, even when the abuse or trauma is no longer occurring, the split or dissociation remains. Integration may take years of intense psychotherapy or may never occur.

The diagnosis of DID is missed more often than it is made. A patient with DID is likely to have had three or more hospitalizations, between three and five mistaken diagnoses and seven years in the mental health system before the diagnosis is made. Reports from or about patients that may lead to ultimate diagnosis of DID include time distortion and blackouts, having been told by others of particular events that happened to the individual; notable changes in the person's behavior during which she calls herself by a different name; a history of severe headaches accompanied by seizures, blackouts, dreams or visions; the use of the term *we* by the individual; the discovery of writings or drawings unrecognized by the patient as his; hearing internal voices; and the appearance of other personalities through hypnosis. (Salama, p. 76).

The best way to learn about DID is through the words of someone who has actually experienced it. The following excerpts from the fascinating book *Living with Your Selves*, by Sandra Hocking, describe such firsthand experience. "All that most people know about multiple personalities is what they read in a book or see in the movies. It's no wonder the public is afraid. What they don't see are the many multiples who have homes, families, jobs, and live a fairly normal life. People with multiple personalities have a psychiatric condition that is caused by severe childhood trauma such as rape, incest, physical torture or ritualistic abuse. Multiplicity is a highly creative and effective method of dealing with pain, trauma, fear and often life-threatening situations. Multiples live complicated lives. Alternate personalities (alters) may come 'out' at inopportune moments and disrupt a conversation. Time loss can be frequent, severe and frightening." (Hocking, p. 1-2)

"Recognition of multiple personalities is simple, yet it is often misdiagnosed. Here are some signs to look for: How much of your childhood and your adult life do you remember? Do you hear conversations going on inside your head? Do you open your mouth in a restaurant and hear yourself order something that you know you hate? Do you say things you have no intention of saying? Do you often feel removed or distant from your surroundings, like you are watching yourself? Do you write in more than one handwriting? Do you have to readjust the seat and mirror every time you get in the car, even though you're the only one who drives it? Do you have flashbacks or nightmares? Do you injure yourself without knowing how, when or why? Have you made the rounds of therapist after therapist, being treated for everything from schizophrenia to borderline-personality disorder, given drugs, sent to hospitals, and nobody can seem to find out what's wrong with you? It sometimes takes years for an accurate diagnosis of multiplicity to be made." (Hocking, p. 9-15)

Conventional treatment of a patient with DID — usually in the form of psychotherapy and hypnosis, sometimes with the addition of medications to alleviate anxiety — averages two to five years. Establishing a safe environment of open communication and trust may be the most important intervention. As you can see by the following case, homeopathic treatment of individuals with DID can also be a lengthy and complicated process and should be undertaken only by a homeopathic practitioner with extensive psychiatric experience; but the rewards can be profound.

"Nobody Really Knows Who I Am"

Grace, thirty-five years old when we first saw her ten years ago, was vivacious and engaging. We treated her intermittently for five years for a variety of complaints, including fibrocystic breast disease. She had a formidable medical history, which included the removal of one breast when she was in her twenties due to cancer (we hadn't discovered this until this past year), a tonsillectomy, three laparoscopies, a tubal ligation and a hysterectomy when in her early thirties, at which time she had been found to have "hundreds of fibroids", and the surgery left only a small portion of one ovary intact. Grace's medical and psychological history has unfolded gradually over the years we have treated her.

For the first five years, Grace came in now and then mostly for physical — often acute — problems, such as hay fever and bladder infections. Although she benefitted from several acute medicines, *Phosphorus* helped her most constitutionally. Now that we have a much better understanding of her, we can go back — even to our first interview with her — to put more of the pieces of the puzzle together. At our first encounter, she told us, "I've had to keep my energy inside. I had a traumatic childhood. A psychologist said I was schizophrenic. At about twelve I started forgetting that I'd bought certain clothes. At twenty-three I realized I had blocks of time for which I couldn't account. I felt different at different times. Like a split personality. Four very distinct people with different names and clothing. I was having terrible nightmares, which I tried to control with drugs. I felt dull. I'm never hungry. I have to set a timer to remind myself to eat. Only now am I beginning to acknowledge and recognize my body. I have balance problems and have to be careful when I stand up. My vision is blurry, starry. I run into things a lot and often don't know where my feet are. I stumble.

"I used to barely eat, from the time I was nineteen or twenty till this year. A can of corn here and there. I couldn't understand why I was so sick. It's like I'm on speed when I don't eat. I get more done. I was bulimic. I'd eat crackers for seven days then binge on ice cream and Ding Dongs. Then I'd vomit. I'd only have a bowel movement once every five days. I stopped being bulimic about a year ago. Bodily functions are new to me. The doctors didn't know what was going on with me partly because they never spoke to each other. I never even admitted to myself that I didn't eat.

"Since I was small, I sleepwalk. Once I cut my head with a knife while I was asleep, though I had no recollection of it. A friend found me. I've found Cheerios in the freezer, my brief-case in the dryer, shoes buried in the flower beds, an iron in the shower. My boyfriend hides the house key at night. Otherwise I'll go out naked. I often wake with a sensation of having walked in the sand. I talk in my sleep, too. I design quilts and paintings between 3 and 5 A.M.

"I have little recollection of my childhood. My sister says I was pitifully obedient. An extremely strict upbringing. My father was a preacher. I flunked lots of classes because I wouldn't talk. We weren't allowed to talk much at home. My brothers don't read or write, and I was the only one to get a high school diploma. Grandma sneaked me into vocational college for a nine-month secretarial program. Now I'm a manager for an international advertising firm.

"When I was about thirty, I attempted suicide several times by taking sleeping pills. Then I tried carbon monoxide. The third time I took pain killers and ended up in the emergency room. Finally I tried psychotherapy. When I get depressed, I become very inward and I just sit for hours. During my hysterectomy I had a near-death experience in which I visited my dead grandmother, who convinced me I had a purpose. It's so hard to establish my boundaries and to identify what I need. Whenever I've been in intimate relationships, I've lost myself. Until three or four years ago I was terrified of everything. I even jumped when the phone rang."

Grace had a wide array of physical complaints, as can be the case with individuals with DID. Her menstrual periods were irregular, with tremendous cramping and ten hours of vomiting. Her hair fell out in clumps. She suffered from recurrent, very painful bladder infections. We treated Grace with several homeopathic medicines over a five-year period with some success. The time came when she was able to reveal herself at a much deeper level, probably because we had more experience and she had more trust in us.

Grace was now able to confide, "My dad didn't like us to talk. I only felt comfortable in the kitchen. I never saw my parents touch. There are periods of time that are just blank. Where I have no recollection of having bought things or done things. My psychiatrist taped one of our sessions. It was my voice but nothing I'd ever say. Something happened when I was very small. My older sister was molested by a neighbor when she was five and I was two and a half."

At this point two things happened: It became clear to us what medicine Grace needed, and the ad agency transferred her to their office in the Netherlands. We transferred her case to an experienced homeopathic physician there. In consultation with us, her physician prescribed homeopathic *Cannabis sativa* (hemp). It is a medicine for people who feel disconnected and have out-of-body experiences whether or not they have any history of taking drugs. This type of escape by splitting off is a common survival mechanism used by children who have been sexually abused. Even when they are safe from the abuse, the personality split persists. There is also an affinity between homeopathic hemp and the urinary tract. Although it is used by practitioners in other parts of the world, this medicine is not available in the United States. Nevertheless, there are other very effective medicines available in this country for patients with DID.

It has been nearly four years since the move and the change of medicines. Grace has suffered from only two bladder infections, each of which has been resolved by use of the *Cannabis sativa*. Grace was able to recover many childhood memories confirming her, and our, suspicion that she was sexually abused. The many elements of her life from which she felt disconnected and distant began to make much more sense. Through twice-yearly doses of the hemp and periodic counseling, all of the personalities except one were successfully integrated. She now has two personalities rather than four. She continues to work for the high-powered advertising agency in Amsterdam and has a very demanding schedule.

In the recent records of her Dutch homeopath, Grace states: "I've been walking straight uphill all my life and now there's a chance to catch my breath. It feels like there's a chance of being whole. These parts of me have had distinct names and personalities, different clothes in my closet. They eat differently. I know now that there's a whole person in there moving toward wholeness. I'm still knowing more and more things that I never knew before. It's like a jigsaw puzzle and the pieces finally fit together. Up close you can see the ridges, but when you stand back it's all one picture. I realize that I felt I could never walk through life without being violated. Now I don't need all the protection. ... I don't have that fear of going over the edge or that I'll black out."

According to her Dutch homeopath, with whom we still correspond regarding Grace's case, she has most recently needed *Phosphorus*, the medicine that helped her years ago.

Grace's journey toward integration is not over. The progress and evolution will continue, as will her homeopathic treatment. This case is a beautiful example of how profoundly homeopathy can work to heal an injured psyche.

26 The Wild World of Hormones

Hormonally Triggered Mental and Emotional Problems

The *H* Word

There is nothing that can make a woman more wild and crazy than *hormones* run amok. What do an adolescent girl starting her menstrual periods, a woman before her periods, a pregnant woman, a postpartum or nursing mother and a woman around menopause have in common? The *H* word: hormones! It is common knowledge that hormonal imbalances can cause fatigue, depression, anxiety, headaches, cramping, abnormal bleeding and vaginal problems. The truth is, a hormonal problem can cause all kinds of symptoms that aren't even listed in any medical textbook. Whatever symptoms a woman already has plus many she did not previously have can be exacerbated during times of hormonal stress.

There is nothing more frustrating for a woman with raging estrogen and progesterone than to be told by a doctor, "Oh, that doesn't have anything to do with hormones. It must be in your head." We have heard women lament that they feel like jumping out of a car prior to their periods or that they have a terrible impulse to kill their newborn child or that they feel as if they are literally jumping out of their skin. Patients out of hormonal balance sometimes refer to themselves as feeling "crazy" or "insane". Anything is possible with unstable hormones.

Hormonal symptoms may vary widely in their intensity, but they are quite prevalent. Surveys have estimated, for example, that as many as 75% of women with regular menstrual cycles experience some symptoms of premenstrual syndrome (PMS). (Steiner, p. 448) An over-whelming number of pregnant and peri- and postmenopausal women suffer from some degree of mental and emotional problems in addition to their physical symptoms.

Homeopathic medicine can be of great benefit for women with all kinds of hormonal problems. We and other homeopaths have seen considerable success in treating PMS, abnormal menstrual cycles and bleeding, morning sickness, post-partum depression, endometriosis, peri- and post-menopausal symptoms, as well as a number of other women's problems. Infertility, depending on the cause and circumstances, can sometimes also be resolved with homeopathy. The following cases speak for themselves.

PMS, Endometriosis and Infertility

Lucy, a twenty-nine-year-old estate agent, sought out homeopathy because of years of suffering from endometriosis, an abnormal growth of uterine tissue outside the uterus. Laparoscopic surgery a year and a half earlier to remove endometrial tissue in the area of the rectum and tailbone had offered only temporary relief of her symptoms. Lucy, infertile for the previous three years, very much wanted a child. She had suffered a miscarriage shortly before beginning homeopathic treatment.

Lucy lamented, "My PMS is ridiculous. I get really aggravated. I feel angry inside. I try not to take it out on others, but I think they're idiots! I get angry even at the way my husband breathes. I snap at him. If he asks me to make a decision, I'm short. I say, 'Don't ask me,' or 'Give me my space.' I'm like this for about ten days every month. I feel better a few hours after my period arrives."

Lucy had a variety of physical symptoms preceding her periods, including extreme water retention, abdominal distention, very tender breasts, a heavy rock-like sensation in her uterus, painful sex, diminished sexual desire and lower-back pain. Lucy also experienced a sharp pain inside her rectum, which worsened when she strained to have a bowel movement.

"I was bulimic for about five years. I didn't have any periods for four of those years. Then, for three years I flowed heavily for three or four days [each month]. I had to put in a tampon every hour or two. My periods are okay now, except my uterus hurts when I put in a tampon. My bulimia lasted from age nineteen to twenty-five. I only ate a small amount of cottage cheese every day, then I vomited at night. From age twenty-five to twenty-six, I drank all day. 1 started drinking when I was seventeen. I drank hard liquor for the first four years, then cheap white wine. I would drink half a gallon in two days."

Lucy was twelve when her parents separated. "It was horrible for me. My world blew apart. There were four of us. That's when I started doing drugs. I quit high school in my senior year and got my high school equivalency certificate. My father is still an alcoholic and my mother came from an alcoholic family. All three of my siblings are in recovery. I've been married five years. I get very jealous. I can be too sympathetic with people. I want to fix it for everyone. Then I berate myself when I can't." Terrified of spiders, Lucy sweated, shook and became paralyzed from seeing a spider on television. She couldn't even talk about spiders. Lucy also had a persistent fear of her husband leaving her.

Lucy's knees were often sore, especially before it rained. She was able to stand in one spot without moving for only five minutes and felt the urge to crack her knees frequently. It was hard for her to sit in movies or a car. Since age twelve, she felt as if her knees didn't fit where they were supposed to. Her wrists had also been weak for much of her life.

Tiny sores inside her nose were an annoyance to Lucy. She often felt chilled, but the heat made her cranky and she couldn't stand saunas or hot baths. An ankle fracture five years before left Lucy with localized pain when it snowed.

We gave Lucy *Calcarea phosphorica* (calcium phosphate), an important medicine for PMS, bone and joint weakness and pain, and dental problems, all related to an inability to assimilate calcium. It is also a medicine for menstrual pain or hormonal problems beginning at puberty, anemia and jealousy; and it is a common homeopathic medicine for knee pain, as well as for incomplete healing of fractures.

At her next visit, five weeks later, Lucy reported that she had had no emotional symptoms before her period. The premenstrual breast tenderness was mild. Sex was pain-free. The shooting rectal pain was gone. The weeks before her period were the easiest in years. "Is this too good to be true?" she asked. Her husband couldn't believe it. He asked in disbelief, "Is it here already?" Lucy did not gain her usual five to seven pounds before her period and had absolutely no premenstrual irritability. Her energy had improved, and her knee pain was somewhat reduced. Considerably less jealous, Lucy felt remarkably better.

When we saw Lucy four months later, her main complaint was nausea from pregnancy! She was very excited about being pregnant — after three years of unsuccessful efforts — but felt terrible. "It's as if I have the flu, but I don't throw up." She had nausea from the moment she woke up in the morning. "I feel like I'm gonna die." The nausea was worse from laughing and the smell of car exhaust, smoke and coffee. Her sexual energy was "zip" since she had become pregnant. In addition, some of Lucy's old symptoms had returned. We repeated the dose of *Calcarea phosphorica* and Lucy sailed through the rest of her pregnancy. She gave birth to an adorable baby girl, whom we have also treated homeopathically.

Lucy has received significant benefit from another homeopathic medicine, *Theridion* (orange spider), which addressed the exquisite sensitivity to noise that was previously noted but had even increased. So painfully affected by noise that it drove her crazy to hear her husband chew at the dinner table, she had also complained of an annoying eczema around and in her ear and a worsening of her premenstrual symptoms, as well as a severe carpal tunnel syndrome of the right wrist. The terrible fear of spiders had also persisted.

Over the past two years Lucy has needed six doses of the *Theridion*. Her PMS symptoms, hypersensitivity to noise, wrist pain, jealousy and eczema have all decreased significantly. She has joined a more successful estate agent's office, enjoys being a mom and is now happily expecting a second child.

Hopelessness, Self-Reproach and Unpredictable Periods

We first met Caroline seven years ago when she sought help for depression, PMS, anger and herpes. A forty-five-year-old computer programmer, she shared with us her history of lifelong depression. The despair was even more exaggerated during holiday seasons. Suicidal thoughts were frequent though she assured us she would never act on the impulses. "I get moody and sullen. My feelings are hurt extremely easily. Everyone says I'm too hard on myself, a perfectionist. I get angry inappropriately. I scream in my car, slam doors or lash out at others. Or I mutter negative comments under my breath like 'You're stupid,' or 'You don't know what you're talking about.' Then I feel mortified and become quiet and unapproachable."

Although she was engaging and witty, Caroline's intimate relationships were few and far between, primarily because she didn't feel good enough. She wondered who would ever want to be with her and preferred no relationship at all to one that was dysfunctional. The belief that she could never do anything right stemmed from childhood, during which time Caroline's mother only criticized and never complimented her. She internalized the powerful message that she was a bad person and aptly described herself as "my own worst enemy". It seemed as if there was some test that she had failed without even knowing she had taken it. Convinced that she would be alone for the rest of her life, Caroline alternated between desiring a companion and closing off any possibility of intimate relationships. Reading proved to be a convenient distraction and escape. Caroline held inside grief over her father's death; and because of her mother's constant deprecation, she had mixed feelings about losing her mother.

A tremendous source of stress was Caroline's job. The victim of a demanding boss, she often worked up to sixty hours a week, including weekends. Aware that her job was taking a terrible toll on her physical and emotional health, Caroline feared that if she quit she wouldn't find another job with similar benefits.

215

But the longer she continued to work at her job, the more worn down and exhausted she became. She felt as if she were stuck in quicksand with no way out. In fact, this is a fitting symbol for how Caroline felt about her life: trapped in her own negativity. The only thing that gave her joy was dancing.

Caroline's periods were unpleasant and unpredictable. All of her emotional symptoms — especially her vulnerability to being offended, her irritability and weepiness — were heightened prior to the onset of her periods. She suffered one miscarriage, for which she continued to grieve. She sometimes bled for twenty-one days of the month and had no idea when her period would stop or start, though her pelvic ultrasounds were normal. Her menstrual flow was often profuse. Physical complaints included recurrent herpes on the lips, periodical sciatica and gas.

The medicine that has helped Caroline immensely is *Sepia*. Mentioned previously, Sepia is one of the foremost homeopathic medicines for treatment of hormonal problems, as well as for irritability, depression, weepiness, mood swings, and for many physical problems, including herpes. Women needing *Sepia* generally love vigorous exercise — particularly dancing. After the first dose, Caroline reported being in a much better emotional state. She had begun to take private dance classes. Her periods were still occurring every eighteen days, but PMS was improved and she felt generally happier, with less of a tendency to dwell on the negative aspects of life. Anger was greatly decreased. Men were on her mind more often and she had a greater desire for sex.

Caroline has continued to need a dose of the medicine every three to six months. Her moods are consistently much more positive, as is her self-image. She has found a job that is less demanding and pays more. Caroline continues to enjoy her dancing and performs occasionally with a group. She left a dingy apartment with a negligent landlord and found a condominium that suits her needs perfectly. She has managed to take one or two vacations a year with friends to places she only dreamed of traveling to previously. Her periods are much more normal, energy is good and irritability is an exception rather than the rule. When she begins to feel on the edge, sharp with people, or excessively hard on herself, a dose of the *Sepia* brings her back into balance. When Caroline does reach menopause, this same medicine is likely to take care of any symptoms that arise.

A Bottomless Pit

Patsy, a forty-year-old part-time receptionist from California, was referred to us by her family-practice physician. "I don't think I've been really happy since my first baby was born. Plus the six miscarriages. I've had a very turbulent relationship with my mother. She tried to commit suicide during my first pregnancy. My parents were abusive. We got hit a lot. It never let up. I was the scapegoat because I was the oldest. I was the child who tried to please my parents. I didn't take a stand to be my own person until I went to college. My insides would just go into turmoil because I was scared to death to do anything wrong. My mother never did like my husband. That's her pattern. She's for ever finding fault with everyone.

"I had a terrible Christmas this year. I cried all through the holidays. Our oldest daughter was having problems with drugs. It was gut wrenching. I just don't know how to smile or have fun around my family. The intense sadness makes me want to cry and never stop. Life feels heavy and dark. Nothing seems to help. There's a black hole in my heart that could never be filled — an intense loneliness. Never a bottom. Like a vacuum. No amount of attention could fill the void.

"I've never felt a part of things, even if I was in a room full of people. I never belonged. I thought I could make it better if I could please everyone. My husband says no matter what he does it's never enough. No matter how much love people gave me, it would just fall out the bottom of the hole, despite my desperate attempts to grasp at it.

"After my first child was born, I just slid into a corner in a fetal position and cried. I could get my feelings hurt and cry for an hour. I still burst into tears at the drop of a hat. The five mis-carriages after my daughter's birth — they said it was because I had a double uterus. I could hardly watch the diaper com-mercials on television without losing it. We visited a friend's baby and I sobbed all the way home. We adopted a son, then I had two more children. I finally decided not to try to get preg-nant again because the doctor said I probably wouldn't survive another birth.

"My periods were never regular and the cramps were really awful. I was so used to not knowing when my period would arrive that I didn't even go for a pregnancy test until I was five months along the first time. Toward the end of that pregnancy, my mother tried to commit suicide. After ten hours of labor, I was still only three centimeters dilated. I started to cry. They ended up doing an emergency C-section. It was a blessing since the cord was wrapped around my baby's neck twice."

Given Patsy's tremendous hormonal ups and downs, it is not surprising that she sank into a postpartum depression. Totally unable to experience spontaneity, everything had to be planned and predicted. Patsy continued to suffer from weepiness, impatience and crankiness premenstrually. She also complained of considerable fatigue and needed to nap every afternoon to make it through the rest of the day.

Quite depressed when we first saw her, Patsy was unable to trust others for fear they would hurt or betray her. She also feared making the wrong decisions in caring for her children or pushing them away, which unfortunately created just the kind of chasm she tried to avert. When we inquired about the funda-mental theme that pervaded her life, she quickly answered that it was a deep sense of being unloved.

In the year and four months that we have treated Patsy, her life has changed impressively for the better, thanks in large part to the homeopathic medicine *Pulsatilla.* She needed four doses during that time and the only new complaint she had was an infected hangnail, which responded beautifully to *Silica* (flint). Within six weeks of beginning homeopathy, Patsy reported feeling "tons better". Happier, more patient and less resentful, she could now stop herself if she started to cry. "I feel like I've wanted to for years and years and years, but I just couldn't get over the hump. I'm not as tired, and my energy is a lot more consistent. My period came on time and I hardly had any cramps at all."

Patsy has continued to flourish. "There are times when I feel so high. I've never felt that way before. I don't cry or get really depressed like before. And I no longer go off on screaming tangents, which my family certainly appreciates. I hardly ever take a nap. I'm doing really well with the kids. A lot more consistency and patience." Patsy has lost fifty pounds following the Zone Diet on our recommendation. She looks younger and more radiant than she has in years. "I keep telling people they have to try homeopathy. It's the best thing that ever happened to me."

The Self-Blame Game

Ann, thirty-or-so pounds overweight, with chestnut brown hair, broke into sobs the moment that she sat in front of us. A stay-at-home mom from Portland, Ann looked more like an unhappy little girl than a mom with her own kids. "I'm really nervous. My hunch is that a lot of my physical problems have been triggered by being a rape survivor since I was seventeen. I grew up in Oregon. I've seemed out of whack all my life. My periods are irregular and I have dark clots. I think a lot of this is because of trying to deal with my emotional issues.

"It's hard to talk about this. I don't like to talk about me. My son really pushes my buttons whenever he wants attention. My husband says I have an attitude all the time. I don't consider him to be one of my stronger supporters. I have a grown daughter who is also a rape survivor. We definitely pass it on from generation to generation. I used to diet and binge, diet and binge. Slimfast, Weight Watchers, Cambridge. You name it and I've tried it. I quit drinking on my own two and a half years ago and I quit smoking five years ago. Food is still a problem. I have good days and bad days.

"I know I'm not in menopause but it's starting. Sometimes I wake really hot in the middle of the night. Mostly what's scaring me is that my PMS is so out of control. I find it disgusting. I get angry and cry and isolate myself. It's no fun. And I would die for chocolate. I even find myself rummaging through the kitchen without realizing it.

"Sometimes I think I was better off before I knew too much about my childhood. I know that my mother wanted a boy and was disappointed that I was a girl. My mother didn't nurse me. She tried but I kept throwing up her milk. Then my brother came along and I was pretty much on the sidelines. I used to dream about my family being ravaged by lions and tigers. I was the only one who escaped. My dad was distant. There wasn't much affection from anyone and my parents were very abusive with each other. My mother used to pick and pick at my dad until it turned into a fistfight. Then it was time to sit down and eat dinner.

"I learned how to stuff a lot of feelings early on. I came to associate food with love and nurturing at a very early age. We weren't allowed to say no to anyone. I was obedient, did quite well academically and spent a lot of time in my room. My younger brother had learning disabilities, so my mother took care of him. He was the household hellion. I was quiet. The little bit of speaking up that I did was squashed. I'd hem up my skirts to make them into miniskirts and my mother would take down the hems while I was at school. I wasn't allowed to date or socialize till I was seventeen. Then I was turned loose.

"A year or two later I was date raped by my first boyfriend. For twenty years I didn't realize what it was. Having been raised a Catholic, the one thing that I valued about myself was taken away without my consent or approval. After all that happened, I figured I was no good. It's hard for me to feel safe. I don't want to be bothered with men. Throughout my life I've played out the victim role. A couple of years after the abuse, I met a guy. Our personalities were like oil and water. He planned to end our relationship but instead he proposed to me. We got married and I got pregnant two weeks later. We stayed together for four years, long enough to have two kids.

"I'm not sure why I got married the second time. It was the dumbest thing I ever did in my life. It lasted for two years. He was a physically abusive alcoholic. My current husband and I have been together twelve years. The relationship seemed to be a lot better when we were both drinking. I know how to fall in love but not how to be in love. I tend to turn things around so that I feel victimized. It's hard for me to feel okay the way I am. If I receive negative criticism, I take it in and believe it, then blame myself. I'm afraid to speak up for myself for fear that I'll be wrong. The bottom line with anything is that I'm not good enough."

Ann described feeling crazy during her hormonal shifts. She also suffered from a variety of physical problems, including an ulcer, a bone spur on the back of her heel, severe menstrual cramps and terrible sinus infections. Since a car accident in her early twenties, she had endured a lot of back pain, particularly muscle spasms in her lower back and hips before her periods. Her neck became so tight prior to her period that she had to ice it three times a day. She also complained of diarrhea and gas and could not tolerate warm, humid weather.

After trying several other medicines with some success, we realized that all of Ann's symptoms pointed toward our giving her *Cimicifuga* (black cohosh), another medicine for sensitive, weepy women with severe menstrual symptoms, spasmodic back and neck pain and a feeling of going crazy. They have a tendency, like the roots of the plant itself, to become entwined, enmeshed, dependent and trapped in intimate relationships.

At Ann's two-month return visit after being given the *Cimicifuga*, she was happy to report that her insane craving for chocolate was gone. She was feeling much better all around until she drank coffee, then relapsed. We repeated the medicine. Each time Ann took the *Cimicifuga*, her menstrual cramping, as well as her neck and shoulder tension, subsided. Her menstrual cycle stabilized at twenty-five days. She began taking computer classes as a move toward possible financial independence. "My husband talks about retiring. I know we can't afford it. I just laugh and don't let him get me down anymore. I'm doing a lot better. I feel more independent. I understand now that I've had a pattern of being drawn to men who put me down.

"Homeopathy has made quite a difference. I'm not as withdrawn. I think more positively. That's a big change. I feel very pleased with how I'm handling boundaries. I'm letting go of other people more. I can stop eating without feeling guilty. Now I often have times when I can't finish my food. I was nuts for chocolate and fats and that is less. I'm finally taking a trip by myself. I'm doing more things like that and not letting my husband be an anchor anymore. Now I enjoy life even if he doesn't."

Ann continued homeopathy for fifteen months after first taking the *Cimicifuga,* during which period she needed several more doses. At that point she discontinued treatment.

PART V

Now That You Know About Homeopathy

27 The Questions People Most Commonly Ask About Homeopathic Treatment

To Help You Better Understand Whether Homeopathy Is for You

We want to make sure that those of you who are new to homeopathy have a good grasp of the basics, so we are including a special chapter with questions and answers.

Can homeopathy really help me with depression?

As you can see from the true cases in our book, many people with depression and other mental and emotional problems can benefit from homeopathic treatment, although each case is individual. If after reading this book you still aren't sure if you're a good candidate for homeopathic treatment, contact an experienced homeopathic practitioner to make sure.

Can I treat myself with homeopathy for depression?

Don't even think about it! You can successfully treat yourself with homeopathy for many first-aid and acute conditions by using a book such as our *Homeopathic Self-Care: The Quick and Easy Guide for the Whole Family* or others that are available. You will be favorably impressed by the rapid results for treatment of bee stings, minor burns, sprains, colds, flus and sore throats. But homeopathic treatment of chronic conditions requires a practitioner with years of study and experience, especially in treating mental and emotional problems. We have written this book to show you that homeopathy may be the answer for you. Now find a qualified practitioner to treat you.

But what if I have a biochemical imbalance?

Homeopathy treats the whole person, bringing into balance every aspect of the individual, neurotransmitters included.

When your organism is in balance mentally, emotionally and physically, you will feel a sense of well-being and your body chemistry will not be a problem.

How will I know if the homeopathic treatment is working?

You will feel happier, have more energy and your thinking will be clearer. Once you have allowed the medicine to act for six to eight weeks, it will be obvious to you whether you feel better. In order for us to be convinced that we have found the best homeopathic medicine, we expect to see at least a 50% — often 70% or greater — improvement that lasts over time. Not only will your depression and anxiety be lessened, so will your physical problems.

What if the first medicine doesn't help me?

Just as with conventional medicine, if the first medicine is not clearly effective, your practitioner will give you a different medicine. Be patient. Healing psychiatric problems is a process.

How long will it take for me to start feeling better?

Some patients feel better within one to several days of beginning treatment, but the most common response time is several weeks. It is best to allow six weeks before evaluating the success of the medicine.

Are there any side effects from homeopathic medicine?

Homeopathic medicines are safe and gentle though they can, at the same time, produce dramatic change. There are no lists of side effects from particular homeopathic medicines as there are with pharmaceutical drugs. You may experience during the first one to three weeks after beginning the medicine a worsening of the symptoms that you already had. This is called an aggravation, is generally short-lived and usually indicates that the medicine that you have been given is correct. If your aggravation is severe, which is rare, or if you develop any new symptoms after taking the medicine, call your homeopath.

How often will I have to take the medicine?

Often a single dose of a homeopathic medicine lasts for months or longer; however there are also times when daily or weekly doses are given. This will depend on your specific complaints and on the style of the practitioner.

If I don't think the medicine is working, why do I have to wait six weeks?

It takes time for the medicine to act and time to evaluate its full effect. Do not rush your practitioner. If you convince him to change medicines sooner than five to six weeks, it is likely to result in confusion rather than cure.

Is it possible that some of the homeopathic medicines are toxic?

Homeopathic medicines are diluted many, many times as they are prepared. They carry the pattern of the original substance but never a physiologic amount sufficient to be poisonous or dangerous, even for pregnant women, infants or the elderly.

Can I begin homeopathic treatment while I am still taking conventional medicine?

Yes. Homeopathy can usually be quite effective despite the use of other medications. You should discuss the specifics with both your homeopathic practitioner and the physician who is prescribing your pharmaceutical drugs.

How long will I need to be treated?

This depends on many factors, including the nature, severity and duration of your complaint. A good rule of thumb is one to two years, or five years for more serious conditions. However, if you are satisfied with homeopathic treatment, you will likely stay with it for life, as have many of our patients.

How often will I need to see my homeopath?

When you first begin treatment, your visits are likely to be scheduled five to eight weeks apart. As you improve, the frequency will diminish to every three to four months or longer.

How expensive is homeopathic treatment?

Your only significant expense will be for office visits, which last approximately one and a half hours for the initial adult appointment and approximately thirty minutes for follow-up appointments. Cost depends on the experience, licensure and location of the practitioner. The expense of the homeopathic medicine is minimal. A year's worth of homeopathic medicine is likely to cost much less than a single month of Prozac.

Is homeopathy covered by insurance?

Although some homeopaths do contract with insurance companies, the majority do not. Many homeopaths choose not to contract with insurers for a variety of reasons, the most fundamental being that insurers do not make adequate provisions for an hour-and-a-half office visit. When insurers understand how effective homeopathy is in keeping people healthy and out of hospitals, they will be eager to include homeopathic practitioners in their plans.

What if I have food or environmental allergies?

Homeopathy treats you as a whole person, allergies and all. We view allergies as the result, rather than the cause, of your being out of balance. As you feel more energy, enthusiasm and calmness with homeopathy, it is very likely that your allergies will improve as well.

How can I find a qualified homeopath in my area?

Unfortunately, availability of well-trained homeopaths is still limited, both in number and geographically. If there are no experienced practitioners of classical homeopathy in your area, some homeopaths, such as ourselves, are willing to treat patients through telephone and video consultations. Long-distance consultations are scheduled and conducted exactly the same as if it were done in person, and results are often as good. Any problems necessitating immediate care or physical or laboratory examination can be handled by a local physician. Whether in person, by telephone or by video, the most important consideration is choosing a qualified and experienced classical homeopath.

28 Homeopathy: Medicine for the Millennium

The Implications of Homeopathy As a Mainstream Medicine

We began our work over twenty years ago with people suffering from mental and emotional illnesses. Many of these unfortunate individuals were destined to lives of unhappiness and permanent inability to function as productive human beings. Some things have changed since that time and others have not. A new family of antidepressants has given the possibility of happiness to some who have never known joy before. But some of the patients who benefit from these drugs do so at the expense of other life-enhancing aspects of a normal life, such as sexual performance. For others, Prozac and the other SSRIs simply don't work. Lithium carbonate has helped to stabilize many patients with bipolar disorder but most need to remain on the medication for life. Conventional medicine still offers no cure for schizophrenia. Mainstream medicine also offers no magic pill to assist recovery from sexual abuse and dissociative identity disorder.

Homeopathy: A Better Alternative?

Our disillusionment long ago with conventional medicine for the treatment of mental illness led us to search for a deeper and more permanent solution. As you can see from the many patients whose true stories appear in this book, we believe that we have found a safe and effective answer for them and many others like them.

Homeopathy, like any therapeutic approach, is not for everyone. Some patients may find it strange and others may be unwilling to give up coffee or camphor. Still others will continue to feel more safe and secure with the conventional approach to medicine. You need to follow your own guidance and intuition about which path is best for you.

228

As we know from the response to our previous book *Ritalin-Free Kids,* many of you who read this book will find new hope and inspiration. Perhaps you have been suffering with depression or anxiety or devastating memories of sexual abuse and have found no help. Maybe you have tried, as has been the case for many of our patients, lots of conventional medications with no dramatic response. Or you might be feeling fine on Prozac but want your sex life back.

Whatever your situation, if after reading this book homeopathy calls to you, we encourage you to contact us, or another experienced practitioner, and to find out for yourself if it is the answer for you. The cost to individual lives and happiness, as well as to society, resulting from mental and emotional illness is tremendous. We firmly believe that the widespread use of homeopathic medicine for patients with mental and emotional problems can dramatically lessen human suffering.

The Merging of Homeopathy into Mainstream Medicine

As further high-quality research is undertaken to prove the efficacy of homeopathic medicine to the scientific community, and as more and more mainstream mental health care practitioners hear from their patients how much these patients have benefited from homeopathic treatment, minds and doors will open. Any approach that is new, different and contrary to the status quo will at first raise eyebrows and doubts. Over time, ideas change and those methods that really work come into acceptance, even if they were scoffed at previously — like the heretical ideas of Copernicus, Newton or Einstein.

At present there is great interest in the field of mind-body medicine, quantum physics and psycho-neuroimmunology. There is much talk about the virtues of treating the whole person and many people are ready for a new type of medicine. There is growing disillusionment with numerous aspects of mainstream healing techniques. Patients may feel dissatisfied with the impersonal, economics-driven medical care. Even the physicians themselves are in some cases unionizing to defend their interests against the HMO (health maintenance organization) conglomerates. Although it is clear that modern medicine is excellent in some areas — such as high-technology diagnosis, microsurgery and trauma management — it is also painfully obvious that conventional medicine is woefully lacking in comprehensive, long-term solutions for cancer and AIDS.

We believe that the time is ripe for homeopathy to attain its rightful place in the health care system. Homeopathic medicine is a safe, gentle, long-lasting, deep-acting and affordable alternative to conventional medicine. And most important of all, as you can see for yourselves from the stories of our patients, it works for many people. May homeopathy flourish over the coming millennium to help millions of people achieve profound healing, happiness and well-being.

Appendix

Recommended Books

Depression, Anxiety, Bipolar Disorder and other Mental and Emotional Problems

Appleton, William. *Prozac and the New Antidepressants.* New York: Plume/Penguin, 1997.

Breggin, Peter, and Ginger R. Breggin. *Talking Back to Prozac: What Doctors Aren't Telling You About Today's Most Controversial Drug.* New York: St. Martin's Press, 1994.

Chodron, Pema. *When Things Fall Apart: Heart Advice for Difficult Times.* Berkeley, CA: Shambhala, 2002.

Elfenbein, Debra, editor. *Living With Prozac and Other Selective Serotonin-Reuptake Inhibitors.* New York: HarperCollins, 1995.

Fieve, Ronald. *Prozac: Questions and Answers for Patients, Family, and Physicians.* New York: Avon Books, 1994.

Hocking, Sandra J., and Company. *Living With Your Selves: A Survival Manual for People with Multiple Personalities*: Rockville, MD: Launch Press, 1992.

Katie, Byron, and Stephen Mitchell. *I Need Your Love: Is It True?* New York City, NY: Crown Publishing Group, 2006.

Katie, Byron. *Loving What Is.* New York City, NY: Three Rivers Press, 2003.

Kramer, Peter. *Listening to Prozac: A Psychiatrist Explores Antidepressant Drugs and the Remaking of the Self.* New York: Penguin, 1993.

Luciani, Joseph. *Self-Coaching: The Powerful Program to Beat Anxiety and Depression.* Hoboken, NJ: Wiley, 2006.

Miklowitz, David. *The Bipolar Disorder Survival Guide: What You and Your Family Need to Know.* New York: Guildford Press, 2010.

Norden, Michael J., M.D. *Beyond Prozac.* New York: Regan Books, 1995.

Papolos, Demitri, M.D., and Janice Papolos. *Overcoming Depression: The Definitive Resource for Patients and Families Who Live with Depression and Manic-Depression*. New York: HarperCollins, 1997.

Ratey, John, and Catherine Johnson. *Shadow Syndromes*. New York: Pantheon, 1997.

Tolle, Eckhart. *A New Earth: Awakening to Your Life's Purpose*. New York City, NY: Dutton Adult, 2005.

Tolle, Eckhart. *The Power of Now: Guide to Spiritual Enlightenment*. Vancouver, B.C.: Namaste Publishing, 1997.

Homeopathy

Bellavite, Paolo, and Andrea Signorini. *Homeopathy: A Frontier in Medical Science*. Berkeley: North Atlantic, 1995.

Castro, Miranda. *Homeopathic Guide to Stress*. New York: St. Martin's Griffin, 1997.

Chappel, Peter. *Emotional Healing with Homeopathy — Treating the Effects of Trauma*. Berkeley, CA: North Atlantic Books, 2003.

Reichenberg-Ullman, Judyth. *Whole Woman Homeopathy: A Safe, Effective, Natural Alternative to Drugs, Hormones, and Surgery*. Edmonds, WA: Picnic Point Press, 2004.

Reichenberg-Ullman, Judyth, and Robert Ullman. *Rage-Free Kids: Homeopathic Medicine for Defiant, Aggressive, and Violent Children*. Edmonds, WA: Picnic Point Press, 2003.

Reichenberg-Ullman, Judyth, and Robert Ullman. *Ritalin-Free Kids: Safe and Effective Homeopathic Medicine for ADD and Other Behavioral and Learning Problems*. Rocklin, CA: Prima, 1996.

Reichenberg-Ullman, Judyth, Robert Ullman and Ian Luepker. *A Drug-Free Approach to Asperger Syndrome and Autism: Homeopathic Care for Exceptional Kids*. Edmonds, WA: Picnic Point Press, 2005.

Sankaran, Rajan. *The Other Song — Discovering Your Parallel Self.* Mumbai, India: Homeopathic Medical Publishers, 2008.

Ullman, Dana. *The Consumer's Guide to Homeopathic Medicine.* New York: Tarcher/Putnam, 1995.

Ullman, Dana. *Homeopathic Family Medicine: Evidence Based eBook.* Berkeley, CA: Homeopathic Educational Services, 2005.

Ullman, Dana. *The Homeopathic Revolution: Why Famous People & Cultural Heroes Choose Homeopathy.* Berkeley, CA: North Atlantic Books, 2007.

Ullman, Robert, and Judyth Reichenberg-Ullman. *Homeopathic Self-Care: The Quick and Easy Guide for the Whole Family.* Rocklin, CA: Prima, 1997.

Ullman, Robert, and Judyth Reichenberg-Ullman. *The Patient's Guide to Homeopathic Medicine.* Edmonds, WA: Picnic Point Press, 1995.

Glossary

affective disorder — a derangement of mood as in depression, anxiety or bipolar disorder

aggravation — a temporary worsening of already existing symptoms after taking a homeopathic medicine

allopathic medicine — a type of medicine that, unlike homeopathy, uses a different — rather than a similar — medicine to heal a set of symptoms

alternative medicine — a natural approach to healing that is nontoxic and safe, which includes homeopathy, naturopathic medicine, chiropractic medicine, acupuncture, botanical medicine, among many other methods of healing

antidepressant — a substance that alleviates depression

antidote — a substance or influence that interferes with homeopathic treatment

antipsychotic — a prescription medication used to treat patients with schizophrenia and other thought disorders

attention deficit disorder (ADD) or **attention deficit hyperactivity disorder (ADHD)** — diagnosis based on a constellation of symptoms that include attention problems, impulsivity and/or hyperactivity

bipolar disorder — a mood disorder, formerly known as manic depression, characterized by episodes of fluctuating moods ranging from depression to mania

case taking — the process of the in-depth homeopathic interview

chief complaint — the main problem that causes a patient to visit a health care practitioner

classical homeopathy — a method of homeopathic prescribing in which only one medicine is given at a time based on the totality of the patient's symptoms elicited in an in-depth interview

combination medicine — a mixture containing more than one homeopathic medicine

235

constitutional treatment — homeopathic treatment based on the whole person, involving an extensive interview and careful follow-up

conventional medicine — mainstream Western medicine

defense mechanism — the aspect of the vital force that maintains health and prevents disease

developmental disability — mental or physical delays in development and maturity due to genetic or congenital abnormalities; previously called mental retardation

dissociative identity disorder (DID) — a dissociative disorder in which two or more distinct persons or personalities inhabit the same body; formerly called multiple personality disorder

DSM-IV — officially recognized diagnostic manual of mental and emotional conditions published by the American Psychiatric Association

FDA — United States Food and Drug Administration

high potency medicines — homeopathic medicines of a 200C potency or higher

homeopathic medicine — a medicine that acts according to the principles of homeopathy

homeopathic practitioner — a practitioner who treats people with homeopathic medicines according to the principles of homeopathic medicine as developed by Samuel Hahnemann

homeopathy — a medical science and art that treats the whole person based on the principle of like cures like

law of similars — the principle of like cures like

low potency medicines — homeopathic medicines of a 30C potency or lower

materia medica — a book that includes individual homeopathic medications and their indications

miasm — an inherited or acquired layer of predisposition

minimum dose — the least quantity of a medicine that produces a change in a person who is ill

modality — those factors that make a particular symptom better or worse

naturopathic physician — a physician who has graduated from a four-year naturopathic medical school and who treats the whole person based on the principle of the healing power of nature

neurotransmitter — a chemical substance, such as serotonin or dopamine, that transmits nerve impulses in the brain and nervous system, affecting thinking, behavior and sensory and motor function

nosode — a homeopathic medicine made from the products of disease

obsessive-compulsive disorder (OCD) — a diagnostic category that includes symptoms of obsessive thought patterns and ritualistic behaviors

panic attack — an episode of extreme anxiety typified by a racing heart, perspiration, hyperventilation, light-headedness, apprehension and fear

phobia —an unreasonable, out of proportion, persistent fear of a specific thing or circumstance

potency — the strength of a homeopathic medicine as determined by the number of serial dilutions and succussions

potentization — the preparation of a homeopathic medicine through the process of serial dilution and succussion

prover — a person who takes a specific homeopathic substance as part of a specially designed homeopathic experiment to test the action of the medicine

provings — the process of testing homeopathic substances in a prescribed way in order to understand their potential curative action on patients

Prozac (fluoxetine) — an antidepressant belonging to the family of SSRIs (selective serotonin-reuptake inhibitors)

relapse — the return of symptoms when a homeopathic medicine is no longer acting

repertory — a book that lists symptoms and the medicines known to produce such symptoms in healthy provers or observed by practitioners in clinical practice among patients

return of old symptoms — the re-experiencing of symptoms from the past after taking a homeopathic medicine, as part of the healing process

Ritalin (methylphenidate) — a stimulant medication commonly used for attention deficit hyperactivity disorder

schizophrenia — a thought disorder characterized by confusion, disorientation, delusions and hallucinations

serotonin — a neurotransmitter in the brain that can affect moods and behavior

simillimum —the one homeopathic medicine that most clearly matches the symptoms of the patient and that produces the greatest benefit

single medicine — one homeopathic medicine given at a time

SSRIs — selective serotonin-reuptake inhibitors, a family of antidepressants that increase levels of serotonin in the brain

state —a n individual's stance in life; how he or she approaches the world

succussion — the systematic and repeated shaking of a homeopathic medicine after each serial dilution

symptom picture — a constellation of all of the mental, emotional, and physical symptoms that an individual patient experiences

thought disorder — derangement of cognitive processes as in schizophrenia

tic disorder — a symptom picture characterized by twitches, jerks and other convulsive or uncontrollable behaviors

totality — a comprehensive picture of the whole person: physical, mental and emotional

vital force — the invisible energy present in all living things that creates harmony, balance and health

Bibliography

Adler U.C., et al. "Homeopathic Individualized Q-potencies versus Fluoxetine for Moderate to Severe Depression: Double-blind, Randomized Non-inferiority Trial." *Evidence-Based Complementary and Alternative Medicine* (2003): 1-8.

Allen, Jane. "Studies Find Serotonin Has a Major Role in Addiction." *Seattle Times* (14 May 1998): A9.

Amadio, P., and L. Cross. "New Drugs for Schizophrenia: An Update for Family Physicians." *American Family Physician* (15 September 1997): 1149-1158.

Andrews, Bernice, and George Brown. "Stability and Change in Low Self-Esteem: The Role of Psychosocial Factors." *Psychological Medicine* 25 (1995): 23-31.

Appleton, William. *Prozac and the New Antidepressants.* New York: Plume/Penguin, 1997.

Begley, Sharon. "Is Everybody Crazy?" *Newsweek* (18 January 1998): 50-53.

Begley, Sharon. "You're OK, I'm Terrific: 'Self-Esteem' Backfires." *Newsweek* (13 July 1998): 69.

Bellavite, Paolo, and Andrea Signorini. *Homeopathy: A Frontier in Medical Science.* Berkeley, CA: North Atlantic, 1995.

Birmaher, Boris, et al. "Childhood and Adolescent Depression: A Review of the Past 10 Years," part 1. *Journal of the American Academy of Child and Adolescent Psychiatry* 35, 11 (November 1996.) 1427-1439.

Blazer, Dan, et al. "The Prevalence and Distribution of Major Depression in a National Community Sample: The National Comorbidity Survey." *American Journal of Psychiatry* 151, 7 (July, 1994): 979-986.

Breggin, Peter, and Ginger Breggin. *Talking Back to Prozac: What Doctors Aren't Telling You about Today's Most controversial Drug.* New York: St. Martin's Press, 1994.

Brown, Donald. "St. John's Wort clinical monograph." *Townsend Letter for Doctors and Patients* (October 1997): 150-151.

Brown-Christopher, Cheryl. "The Growing Depression Phenomenon." *Journal of Longevity Research* 3, 6 (1997): 42-43.

Chambers, Christina, et al. "Birth Outcomes in Pregnant Women Taking Fluoxetine." *New England Journal of Medicine* 335 (3 October 1996): 1010-1015.

Chopra, Deepak. *Quantum Healing.* New York: Bantum, 1989.

Ciabattari. Jane. "The Most Popular Prescription Drugs." *Parade* (12 July 1998): 16.

Cipriani, A., et al. "Comparative efficacy and acceptability of 12 new-generation antidepressants: a multiple-treatments meta-analysis." *Lancet,* 353 (28 February 2009): 746-758.

"Clam Dunk." *People* (13 July 1998): 79.

CNN Health.com. "CDC: Antidepressants most prescribed drugs in U.S." *CNN health.com.* (9 July 2007).

Convey, Eric. "Mass. General Disciplines. Three Psychiatrists." *Boston Business Journal,* (1 July 2011).

Crowley, Mary. "Do Kids Need Prozac?" *Newsweek* (20 October 1997): 73-74.

Cunningham, Lynn. "Depression & Anxiety in the Primary Care Setting." *Comprehensive Therapy,* 23,6 (1997): 400-406.

Davenas, F., et al. "Human Basophil Degranulation Triggered by Very Dilute Antiserum Against IgE." *Nature* 333 (30 June 1988): 816-818.

Elfenbein, Debra, ed. *Living With Prozac and Other Selective Serotonin-Reuptake Inhibitors.* New York: HarperCollins, 1995.

Emoto, Masaru. *Messages from Water.* Tokyo: Sunmark Publishing Co. Ltd., 1999.

Emoto, Masaru. *Love Thyself: Messages From Water, III.* Carlsbad, CA: Hay House, 2006.

Ernst, E. "St. John's Wort, an Antidepressant? A systemic, criteria-based review." *Phytomedicine* 2 (1995): 67-71.

"Examining Atypical Antipsychotic Use in Children" *Physicians Weekly,* (14 June 2011): No. 23.

Fieve, Ronald. *Prozac: Questions and Answers for Patients, Family, and Physicians.* New York: Avon Books, 1994.

Finkelhor, David, and Lucy Berliner. "Research on the Treatment of Sexually Abused Children: A Review and Recommendations." *Journal of the American Academy of Adolescent Psychiatry* 34, 11 (November 1995): 1408-1423.

Fournier, J.C., et al. "Antidepressant Drug Effects and Depression Severity: A Patient Level Meta-analysis." *JAMA*, 303, 1 (2010): 47-53.

Gaby, Alan. "Drugging Our Children." *Townsend Letter* 336 (July 2011): 107.

Gibbons R.D., et al. "Early evidence on the effects of regulators' suicidality warnings on SSRI prescriptions and suicide in children and adolescents". *The American Journal of Psychiatry 164, 1* (2007): 1356–1363.

"Girls Are Depressed Because They Worry Too Much." *Seattle Times* (15 August 1998): A3.

Hahnemann, Samuel. *Organon of Medicine*, sixth edition (translation). Boston: Tarcher, 1982.

Harris, Gardiner. "Use of Antipsychotics in Children Is Criticized." *N.Y. Times* (18 November 2008): A20.

Hegarty, James D. "Suicidal and Violent Behavior Associated with the Use of Fluoxetine." Drugs and Devices Information Line Harvard School of Public Health, *http://www.hsph.harvard.edu/organizations/DDIL/ddil.html*, 1995.

Hirschfeld, Robert. "Panic Disorder: Diagnosis, Epidemiology, and Clinical Course." *Journal of Clinical Psychiatry 57*, suppl. 10 (1996): 3-10.

Hocking, Sandra J., and Company. *Living with Your Selves: A Survival Manual for People with Multiple Personalities.* Rockville, MD: Launch Press, 1992.

"Is It the Pimples or the Pills?" *Newsweek* (March 1998): 64.

Jamison, Kay Redfield. "Manic-Depressive Illness and Creativity." *Scientific American, Mysteries of the Mind*, Special Issue Vol. 7, no. 1 (1997): 44-49.

Jonas, et al. "A Critical Overview of Homeopathy." *Annals in Internal Medicine*, 138, 2003: 393-399.

Kah, M., and A. Michael. "Major Depression in Children and Adolescents." *British Journal of Hospital Medicine* Vol. 55, no. 1/2 (1996): 57-61.

Katerndahl, David. "Panic Attacks and Panic Disorder." *Journal of Family Practice* 213043, 3 (September 1996): 275-282.

Kessler R.C., et al., Prevalence, severity, and comorbidity of twelve-month DSM-IV disorders in the National Comorbidity Survey Replication (NCS-R). *Archives of General Psychiatry*, 62, 6 (June 2005): 617-627.

Kleijnen, Paul, Paul Knipschild and Gerben ter Riet. "Clinical Trials of Homoeopathy." *British Medical Journal* 302 (9 February 1991): 316.

Lemonick, Michael. "The Mood Molecule." *Time* (29 September 1997): 74-82.

Leviton, R. "Schizophrenia: Healing the Divided Self with Nutrients." *Alternative Medicine* 24 (July 1998): 42-49.

Linde, Klaus, et al. "Are the Clinical Effects of Homeopathy Placebo Effects? A Meta-Analysis of Placebo-Controlled Trials." *Lancet* 350 (1997): 834-843.

Longo, Lance, and Bradley Johnson. "Addiction: Part 1. Benzodiazepines — Side Effects, Abuse Risk and Alternatives." *American Family Physician*, (April 2000): 2121-2130.

Maddox, J. "When to Believe the Unbelievable." *Nature* 333 (30) (1988): 787.

Manolis, Deane. "The Perils of Prozac." *Minnesota Medicine* Vol. 78 (January 1995): 19-23.

Motsinger, et al. "Use of Atypical Antipsychotic Drugs in Patients with Dementia." *American Family Physician*, (1 June 2003): 2335-2341.

Myers, David, and Diener Meyers. "The Pursuit of Happiness." *Scientific American, Mysteries of the Mind, Special Issue* Vol. 7 (1997): 40-43.

NIMH. "Bipolar Disorder Among Children." *NIMH,* reviewed 29 July 2010. http://www.nimh.nih.gov/statistics/1BIPOLAR_CHILD.shtml.

NIMH. "Anxiety Disorders." *NIMH,* reviewed 2 December 2010. http://www.nimh.nih.gov/health/publications/anxiety-disorders/complete-index.shtml.

NIMH. "Major Depressive Disorder Among Adults." *NIMH,* reviewed 29 July 2010. http://www.nimh.nih.gov/statistics/1MDD_ADULT.shtml.

Nishizawa, S., et al. "Differences Between Males and Females Rates of Serotonin Synthesis in Human Brain." *Proceedings of the National Academy of Science* 94 (May 1997): 5308-5313.

"Not Just for Anxiety Anymore." *Newsweek* (6 October 1997): 8.

Null, Gary. "Prozac, Eli Lilly and the FDA." *Townsend Letter For Doctors* (February-March 1993): 178-182.

Okie, Susan. "Wild About Wort: Ancient Herb Gaining Popularity as a Treatment for Depression." *Washington Post* as reprinted in the *Seattle Times* (19 November 1997): E2-3.

Olfson, Mark and Steven C. Marcus."National Patterns in Antidepressant Medication Treatment." *Archives of General Psychiatry,* Vol 66(8) (Aug 2009): 848-856.

Papolos, Demitri, and Janice Papolos. *Overcoming Depression: The Definitive Resource for Patients and Families Who Live with Depression and Manic-Depression.* New York: HarperCollins, 1997.

Pert, Candace. "Letters to the Editor." *Time* (20 October 1997): 8.

Pincus, Harold, et al. "Prescribing Trends in Psychotropic Medications: Primary Care, Psychiatry, and Other Medical Specialties." *Journal of the American Medical Association* Vol. 279, no. 7 (18 February 1998): 526-531.

Prozac advertisement in *Newsweek* (21 July 1997): 2.

Reuters. "Prozac Is Found to Help Clams in Spawning." *New York Times* (17 April 1998): A19.

Rapaport, Jennifer. "Shaking the Blues." *Natural Health* (July-August 1997): 99-101, 159-166.

Ratey, John, and Catherine Johnson. "Shadow Syndromes." *Seattle Times* (22 August 1997): F1-2.

Reichenberg-Ullman, Judyth, and Robert Ullman. *Ritalin-Free Kids: Safe and Effective Homeopathic Medicine for ADD and Other Behavioral and Learning Problems.* Rocklin, CA: Prima, 1996.

Reilly, David, et al. "Is Evidence for Homoeopathy Reproducible?" *Lancet* Vol. 344 (10 December 1994): 1601.

Ritter, M. "Scientists Close in on Manic-Depression Gene Locations." *Seattle Times* (3 June 1998): A15.

Sahentara, Amelia Jo. *Free To Love: A Journey of Healing.* Manzanita, OR: Akawa Publishing, 1997.

Salama, A. Aziz. "Multiple Personality Disorder." *Journal of the American Medical Association of Georgia* Steven C. Vol. 84 (February 1995): 75-79.

Sasson, Yehuda, et al. "Epidemiology of Obsessive-Compulsive Disorder: A World View." *Journal of Clinical Psychiatry* 58, suppl. 12 (1997): 7-10.

Schweizer, Edward, and Karl Rickels. "Placebo Response in Generalized Anxiety: Its Effect on the Outcome of Clinical Trials." *Journal of Clinical Psychiatry* 58, suppl. 11 (1997): 30-38.

Steiner, Meir. "Premenstrual Syndromes." *Annual Review of Medicine* 48 (1997): 447-455.

Strauch, Barbara. "Prozac- Type Drugs Being Given to Kids: Drug Firms Want FDA Endorsement." *New York Times* as reprinted in the *Seattle Times* (10 August 1997): A1, A19.

"2010 Top 200 Generic Drugs by Total Prescriptions." http://drugtopics.modernmedicine.com/Pharmacy *Facts and Figures*

Ullman, Dana. *The Consumer's Guide to Homeopathic Medicine.* New York: Tarcher/Putnam, 1995.

Ullman, Dana. *Homeopathic Family Medicine: Connecting Research to Quality Homeopathic Care.* Berkeley: Homeopathic Educational Services, 2011. E-book.

Ullman, Robert, and Judyth Reichenberg-Ullman. *The Patient's Guide to Homeopathic Medicine.* Edmonds, WA: Picnic Point Press, 1995.

Van Wassenhoven, M., "Priorities and Methods for Developing the Evidence Profile of Homeopathy: Recommendations of the ECH General Assembly and XVIII Symposium of GIRI." *Homeopathy* 94 (April 2005):94, 107-124.

Warshaw, M.G., and M.B. Keller, "The Relationship Between Fluoxetine Use and Suicidal Behavior in 654 Subjects with Anxiety Disorders." *Journal of Clinical Psychiatry* 57, 4 (1996): 158-166.

Web MD, http://www.webmd.com/bipolar-disorder/guide/bipolar-disorder-symptoms-types.

"Women Produce Less of Key Mood-Control Chemical Than Men." *Washington Post* as reprinted in the *Seattle Times* (13 May 1997): A10.

Wilson, Duff. "Side Effects May Include Lawsuits." *New York Times* (2 October 2010): BU1.

Xu, J. et al. *"Deaths: Preliminary Data for 2007".* National Vital Statistics Reports 58 (1): 29–30. http://www.cdc.gov/nchs/data/nvsr/nvsr58/nvsr58_01.pdf.

Index of Remedies

Index

E

ear infections 128, 144, 180
eating disorders 92, 207, 213, 219
 – *See also* anorexia; bulimia; compulsive eating
eating well 71
eczema xiii-xiv, 189-191, 196, 214
Edith (case study) 97
Effexor (venlafaxine) 6, 14, 25, 51, 125
Eli Lilly 8, 29, 125-126
endometriosis 212
estrogen 4, 30, 95, 211
eucalyptus 61
exercise 71
eye movement desensitization reprocessing (EMDR) 202

F

fantasy life 146, 187
fear
 – of butterflies/moths 177
 – of castration 199
 – of flying 141, 142
 – of heights 114, 116, 144, 151, 177
 – of spiders 213
 – *See also* anxiety
fenfluramine 18
fibromyalgia 43, 196
fluvoxamine
 – *See* Luvox
Fong, Peter 16
Food and Drug Administration (FDA) 5, 18, 24-27, 125, 134
 – homeopathic medicine regulated by 41
food cravings
 – *See* eating disorders
forgiveness 70

fraternal twin studies 4
Freddie (case study) 187
friends 69

G

genital mutilation fear 199
George (case study) 198
God 85, 102-103, 161-162, 189-191
Goethe, Johann 158
good company 69
 – *See also* relationships
good people/bad things 67
Grace (case study) 206
gratitude 70
grief 82
guilt 83
 – sexual 126, 190, 198
Gwen (case study) 183

H

Hahnemann, Samuel 36, 40-41
Haldol (haloperidol) 165, 188
hallucinations 61, 146, 157, 182, 188
hallucinogenic drug use 193
 – *See also* drug abuse
Handel, George Friederich 158
happiness
 – articles on 2
 – Prozac and 31
 – self-love and 118
Harborview Medical Center 195
Hashimoto's thyroiditis 89
headaches xiii, 87, 112, 156, 160, 171, 183-184
healing relationships 70
hectic lives 100
Heilpraktikers 48
Helen (case study) 200

Homeopathy: A Frontier in Medical
   Science (Bellavite and Signorini) 44
honesty 61, 68, 150
hormonal problems 211
Hughes, Howard 169
humor 68
hypo-chondriasis 170
hypoglycemia 139

I

identical twin studies 4
immunoglobulin antibody (IgE) 44
impulsive behavior 158
incest 115, 205
incontinence 98, 116, 183-186
Inderal (propranol) 30
infertility 212
inositol 47
insomnia 11, 84, 116, 134, 137, 144, 160
insurance coverage 227
Irene (case study) 145
isolation 110

J

Jack (case study) 149
Jackie (case study) 135
Japanese school-aged boys 125
Jeremy (case study) 129
Jimmy (case study) 154
Johnson, Catherine 3
Johnson, Dr. Samuel 169
Joyce (case study) 165

K

Kelsey (case study) 120
kindness 68
kleptomania 170
Klonopin (clonazepam) 158

L

Lancet, The 43
laughter 68
law of similars 37, 236
Leanne (case study) 110
learning disabilities 176, 180
   – See also attention deficit hyper-
      activity disorder
life energy (vital force) 56
Lily (case study) 161
Lincoln, Abraham 158
liquid crystals formation 42
lithium 15, 31, 79, 158-166, 228
Living with Your Selves (Hocking)
   205
lonliness 110
loss/grief 82
love 65
Lowell, Robert 158
LSD 192, 193
Lucy (case study) 212
Luvox (fluvoxamine) 6, 14-18
lying 68

M

Mahler, Gustav 158
manic depression
   – See bipolar disorder
Max (case study) 100
McGill University 6
medicine
   – See conventional medicine;
      holistic medicine; homeopathic
      medicine
Meg (case study) 102
Melanie (case study) 105
melatonin 47
menstrual symptoms 211

About the Authors

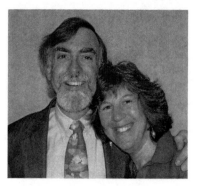

Judyth Reichenberg-Ullman, N.D., M.S.W., and Robert Ullman, N.D., are licensed naturopathic physicians and board-certified diplomats of the Homeopathic Academy of Naturopathic Physicians. Dr. Reichenberg-Ullman received a doctorate in naturopathic medicine from Bastyr University in 1983, and a master's degree in psychiatric social work from the University of Washington in 1976. Dr. Ullman received his naturopathic medical degree from the National College of Naturopathic Medicine in 1981, and completed graduate coursework in psychology at Bucknell University in 1975. Both doctors had extensive experience in conventional mental health settings prior to their medical training. Dr. Reichenberg-Ullman is the past President of the International Foundation for Homeopathy, and past Vice President of the Homeopathic Academy of Naturopathic Physicians. Dr. Ullman is past Vice President of the International Foundation for Homeopathy. The doctors are authors of seven books on homeopathic medicine, including the best-selling *Ritalin-Free Kids*. They have been columnists for the *Townsend Letter* since 1990, and have taught throughout the U.S. and internationally.

Drs. Reichenberg-Ullman and Ullman practise at The Northwest Center for Homeopathic Medicine in Edmonds, Washington. As classical homeopaths, they specialize in treating adults with mental and emotional problems, and children with behavioral, learning, and developmental problems, as well as their general homeopathic practice. Dr. Reichenberg-Ullman also specializes in natural women's health care.

They have studied intensively with Dr. Rajan Sankaran, (Sensation Method) of Mumbai, India, since 1993, and with Dr. Divya Chhabra since 2000. Drs. Reichenberg-Ullman and Ullman are very comfortable and experienced treating patients by telephone and video consultation, as well as in person. Many of their patients live throughout the U.S. and abroad. Dr. Reichenberg-Ullman is fluent in Spanish. The couple lives in Langley, Washington, on Whidbey Island, and in Pucon, Chile, with their golden retrievers, cats, chickens and sheep.

Contacting the Authors:

To become a patient or to reach the doctors, call (425) 774-5599.
The office email address is nchmclinic@gmail.com.
To reach Dr. Reichenberg-Ullman, use drreichenberg@gmail.com.
To reach Dr. Robert Ullman, use drbobullman@gmail.com.
Their website is www.healthyhomeopathy.com.

Our Books and Kits

Books can be ordered through our website at:www.healthyhomeo-pathy.com. For additional questions, please email nchmclinic@gmail.com or call (425) 774-5599. We offer discounts on orders of 5 or more books/kits.

The Homeopathic Treatment of Depression, Anxiety, Bipolar Disorder, and Other Mental and Emotional Problems: Homeopathic Alternatives to Conventional Drug Therapies

280 pages. (2012. Revised edition of *Prozac Free*). Explores the homeopathic treatment of depression, anxiety, bipolar disorder, mood swings, phobias, panic disorder, multiple personality disorder, schizophrenia, and hormonally-induced mental and emotional problems. Includes nearly forty successfully-treated cases from our practice. $22.95.

Ritalin-Free Kids: Safe and Effective Homeopathic Medicine for ADHD and Other Behavioral and Learning Problems

300 pages. (Revised editions in 2000 and 2012). Revised edition. Foreword by Edward Hallowell, MD, author of *Driven to Distraction*. Bestseller—over 60,000 copies sold. Demonstrates that homeopathy can be very effective with children and adults with ADHD, learning disabilities, anger, depression, fears, autism, and developmental delays. $22.95.

Rage-Free Kids: Homeopathic Medicine for Defiant, Aggressive and Violent Children

320 pages. (1999). Focuses on the causes, conventional approach, and homeopathic treatment of children with ADHD, oppositional-defiant disorder, conduct disorder, and abused children. Includes nearly thirty fascinating cases from our practice, as well as practical tips to deal with your angry child. $19.95.

A Drug-Free Approach for Asperger Syndrome and Autism: Homeopathic Care for Exceptional Kids

290 pages. (2005). Foreword by Bernard Rimland, M.D. Discusses the symptoms and prevalence of Asperger Syndrome and autism.

Includes seventeen cases, from our practice, of children on the autism spectrum, who have benefited from homeopathic treatment. Compelling comments of parents of ASD children whom we have treated. $22.95.

Homeopathic Self-Care: The Quick and Easy Guide for the Whole Family

325 pages. (1997). In-depth instructions for self-treating 70 acute conditions such as colds, flu, sore throats, burns, insect bites, bladder infections, motion sickness, and many others. Homeopathic as well as naturopathic recommendations. Icons, charts. The clearest and most easy-to-use homeopathic self-care book available. $21 (Book and companion kit $120.

Homeopathic Self-Care Home Medicine Kit

Companion kit to *Homeopathic Self-Care*. Contains the 50 most commonly prescribed medicines as included in our book. $105.

Whole Woman Homeopathy: A Safe. Effective, Natural Alternative to Drugs, Hormones, and Surgery

430 pages. (2000). A practical, user-friendly book that offers specific information on self-treating 20 women's conditions such as bladder infections, morning sickness, and vaginal infections with naturopathic as well as homeopathic self-treatment. Explains when you need a homeopath. Includes many successful cases. $22.95.

The Patient's Guide to Homeopathic Medicine: Everything You Need to Know to Make the Most of Your Treatment

113 pages, (1995). Practical, easy-to-understand book for patients about homeopathic treatment. Includes answers to the most commonly asked questions. $12.

Mystics, Masters, Saints, and Sages: Stories of Enlightenment

289 pages, Conari, 2001. Foreword by The Dalai Lama. Self-told accounts of awakening of 34 great teachers past and present, from diverse traditions. $16.95.

262

CPSIA information can be obtained at www.ICGtesting.com
Printed in the USA
LVOW06s1704030314

375862LV00017B/701/P